Lotus of the Heart

*Living Yoga for Personal Wellness
and Global Survival*

Tracey Winter Glover

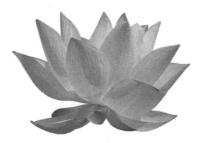

Lantern Books • New York
A Division of Booklight Inc.

2016
Lantern Books
128 Second Place
Brooklyn, NY 11231
www.lanternbooks.com

Copyright © 2016 Tracey Winter Glover

Notice: This book is intended as a reference volume only, not as a medical manual. The information given here is designed to help you make informed decisions about your health. It's not intended as a substitute for any treatment that may have prescribed or recommendations given by your health care provider. If you suspect that you have a medical problem, we urge you to seek competent medical help.

Printed in the United States of America

Library of Congress Cataloging-in-Publication Data

Names: Glover, Tracey Winter, author.
Title: Lotus of the heart : living yoga for personal wellness and global survival
    / Tracey Winter Glover.
Description: New York : Lantern Books, 2016.
Identifiers: LCCN 2015041786 (print) | LCCN 2015049184 (ebook) | ISBN
9781590565339 (pbk. : alk. paper) | ISBN 9781590565346 (epub)
Subjects: LCSH: Detoxification (Health) | Hatha yoga—Therapeutic use.
Classification: LCC RA784.5 .G635 2016 (print) | LCC RA784.5 (ebook) |
    DDC
613.7/046—dc23
LC record available at http://lccn.loc.gov/2015041786

Lotus of the Heart

OF RELATED INTEREST

Ruth Lauer-Manenti
An Offering of Leaves
Foreword by David Life

Ruth Lauer-Manenti
Sweeping the Dust
Foreword by Sharon Gannon

Ruth Lauer-Manenti
Fell in Her Hands

Mark Whitwell
Yoga of Heart
The Healing Power of Intimate Connection

Will Tuttle
The World Peace Diet
Eating for Spiritual Health and Social Harmony

"All things are one."
—**Heraclitus** (500 B.C.E.)

"Nothing in this world purifies like spiritual wisdom."
—**Lord Krishna** in the *Bhagavad Gita*

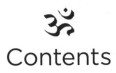

Contents

ॐ
Introduction

All things are connected. What we do to ourselves, we do to the planet. What we do to other living beings, we do to ourselves. This is the secret to discovering the purity, health, and wellness we seek. True health is not just the absence of physical disease in the body but a state of balance within, a capacity for joy and an ability to live life to its fullest. Real wellness implies happiness, peace, dignity, and the sort of deep confidence and ease that come from being in touch with our most authentic selves. When we awaken to our interconnection with all life, we see that the path that leads to personal wellness is the same that leads to the well-being of all living beings and our fragile living planet. Our fates are not separate because we are not separate.

As a society, all of us seem to feel toxic, cloudy, and somehow impure. This makes perfect sense in a world where it's inevitable we will be exposed to toxins no matter the lengths we go to protect ourselves. We are exposed to toxins in our household products, in the air we breathe, the water we drink, and the foods we consume. Even our own miraculous bodies are toxin factories when stressed, as most of us are. As a country, we are really sick. Either we ourselves have personally experienced some frightening illness or someone we love has. We're scared, and we want to be well.

True wellness, however, won't come from a miracle drink, a juice fast, a weekend detox, or any physical cleanse, however rejuvenating these may be. True health will only come with a fundamental overhaul of the way we approach life. The good news is that there is an integrated approach to living that can bring us into the state of health we seek. It begins with the recognition that we are multidimensional beings.

We are more than our physical bodies, and true health cannot be achieved by focusing exclusively on cleansing the physical body.

Keeping the body pure is an essential component of good health. What we eat and how we care for these bodies is of undeniable importance. However, no matter how "pure" the body is, if the heart, the soul, or the psyche is neglected, we can juice and detox and colon cleanse ourselves without end, and we will never find the purity or health we seek. For all of the toxins we consume with the physical body, we consume far more through the senses of the mind and the heart. That for which we as a society seem to be desperately groping cannot be found through bodily purification practices alone.

The truth is that we've become ill as a result of the choices we make as individuals and as a society. This isn't cause for despair or self-recrimination. It is, in fact, reason for hope. We can learn to make wiser choices. We can go to the source of our choices, to the mind itself, and begin our cleansing there. We can clear the habitual thought patterns that drive us to the persistent actions that create the need for the detox in the first place.

Lotus of the Heart uses yogic and other Eastern philosophies, including key teachings of the Buddha, as a framework for this retraining. Ultimately, as we learn to control the mind, we come to understand that at the core of our being we are already pure, perfect, and whole. In yogic terms, we are "Divine," a word I will use throughout this book to refer to our own basic goodness, our own highest potential, and that same essence dwelling in all sentient beings. No matter what we do, that purity remains at our core. Our work is to shed all that blocks us from that natural state in which we can live in harmony not just with ourselves but with all life.

One of the most serious symptoms of our current societal sickness is our disconnection from nature. We don't see ourselves as being a part of nature. We don't see ourselves as a small fiber of nature, but rather as her dominator. We don't see that all parts are interconnected, that as we are poisoning our planet, we are simultaneously poisoning ourselves. We are currently in the midst of the sixth greatest extinction in Earth's long history. Unlike previous extinctions, this one is directly caused by humanity: from hunting and fishing, clear-cutting of forests, climate change, pesticide use—the list goes on. There isn't just one thing we're doing wrong. The problem is systemic. Our entire approach to living on this planet is fundamentally destructive. We must transform the way we relate to Earth or she will perish, and we will go with her.

Eastern philosophies like Buddhism, Hinduism, Yoga, and Jainism, which share a common view that we are part of a whole and that we are connected with all other beings, can offer us a solution both to our own personal disease and that of the planet. They teach us that real wellness depends on our ability to see and to respect the whole of life. They teach that the ultimate purification is wisdom, and the ultimate wisdom is this interconnection with all life.

According to these wisdom traditions, "right diet" is central to health and wellness. What is "right" isn't so much a moral judgment as it is an objective observation about what sorts of behaviors bring us into balance and harmony with ourselves, with ultimate truth, and with the truth of interconnection. The practices and way of life that bring us into harmony with the Divine within ourselves and with all life, from other human beings and the nonhuman animals to all of nature, bring us into a state of health and happiness and are therefore considered "right." Those habits and practices that lead to disharmony and disease are seen as "wrong."

The Eastern view of right diet accords with modern nutrition and modern environmental science, too. Integrating both the ancient and modern perspectives gives us a spiritual and practical framework within which to achieve health, wholeness, and purity. If we live clean and avoid ingesting toxins in the first place, we won't need to detox or cleanse.

Rooted in deep spiritual truths and solid modern science, *Lotus of the Heart* is more than just a manual for cleansing or detoxing the body. It provides a complete practical architecture for a good life. A mostly Eastern-influenced philosophy and spirituality provide the foundation for a range of applied practices including deep breathing exercises, meditations, and a complete yoga practice. Plus, I integrate traditional Eastern wisdom with modern Western science as a basis for understanding disease prevention, nutrition, and environmental sustainability. Ultimately, this book makes the case that the greatest medicine is to live in harmony with the laws of the universe, of which we are an integral part. I hope this book can help us see the very tangible ways in which we are all connected to one another and to all life. With this understanding, we can begin to see the path to personal and planetary healing, wellness, and a life well lived that lies before us, ready to support and nurture us every step of the way. ❁

1

Yoga as a System of Purification

Yoga is an ancient system of purification that works from the outside in and the inside out and is ultimately believed to bring us into a state of health on the physical, mental, and spiritual planes. Rather than providing an exhaustive compendium of yogic practices, this book will focus on some key teachings and practices that can help us connect to all life and enable us to find harmony. They will allow us to understand ourselves more fully, break through the obstacles we place in our own way, and liberate ourselves.

The word *yoga* means "union," or "to yoke or bind." The term is generally used to refer to a range of physical, mental, and spiritual practices originating in India that are designed to help us find the balance that comes from being in tune with our own Divine nature. Yoga has a long history, going back as far as five thousand years ago. Much of the history remains mysterious and likely bears little resemblance to most of what we Westerners call "yoga" today. In about 500 B.C.E., the sage Patanjali memorialized a yogic system comprised of eight major components or "limbs." These include the *yamas* (ethical proscriptions), *niyamas* (ethical prescriptions), *asana* (physical postures), *pranayama* (breath control), *pratyahara* (sense withdrawal), *dharana* (one-pointed concentration), *dhyana* (meditation), and *samadhi* (spiritual absorption). This is what is considered classical or *raja* (royal) yoga. These practices are described in his *Yoga Sutras*, which forms the foundational text of *Raja Yoga*.

The most recognizable of the eight limbs to many of us in the West is asana, or the physical posture. In the early days of yoga, the physical practices were probably a fairly minor component of a system ultimately designed to lead practitioners into deep meditation, through which they hoped to attain enlightenment or samadhi, complete absorption in the Divine. The physical postures were seen primarily as a tool to prepare and condition the body for meditation with this final goal in mind.

Whereas Eastern cultures have a rich history of meditation practices, we in the West have a very limited and sometimes difficult relationship with meditation. There is a long history of persecution of those Christian mystics who discovered that they didn't need priests to connect with God but looked within to experience the Divine directly. So when yoga came west, we absorbed the teachings in a particularly Western way, placing disproportionate emphasis on the physical postures and de-emphasizing the remainder of the teachings—including the ethical teachings and the more mystical, introverting practices such as sense withdrawal (pratyahara), gradual stages of meditation (dhyana and dharana), and finally union with the Divine (samadhi).

Westerners have this tendency to deconstruct the whole and isolate the parts. We can see this throughout our health-care system, from the way we treat the body as separate from the mind to the way we treat symptoms of disease through pills and surgeries, without addressing the underlying lifestyle issues that are causing so many of our problems. Real, enduring health lies in a more holistic approach. And yoga offers us such a holistic approach. But in order to obtain the full benefits of yoga, and the purity, peace, and bliss that yoga promises is our true nature, we must go beyond simply toning the body through asana and the other physical purification practices. We must go deeper and recognize that yoga is a system of practices for the mind, body, and soul.

Purity of Mind, Speech, and Body *(Saucha)*

According to the path of raja yoga, *saucha*—or "purity" in mind, speech, and body—is the foremost of the ethical prescriptions, or niyamas, which constitute the second limb of yoga.[1] We can approach each aspect separately, though in truth, of course, they are all connected.

Probably the most straightforward aspect of saucha is purity of the physical body. This comes from a range of practices including eating a pure diet (discussed at length below) and keeping our bodies clean both externally and internally through the practice of asana, pranayama, and other cleansing practices called *kriyas* (also discussed below).

The practice of saucha also includes maintaining a clean and organized external environment. Keeping a clean and organized home, car, or office space can help us achieve purity in other aspects of our lives as well. When our physical spaces are cluttered, our minds tend to be cluttered as well. Maintaining simplicity and order in our external environments helps us bring order to our minds. Just as an unhealthy body is a distraction from our spiritual practice, a disorganized living environment is an obstacle to the clarity and purity of mind we seek.

The people with whom we interact are an important aspect of our environment as well. While we work toward a life of peace and balance, our path will be much smoother if we surround ourselves with others working toward the same ends. If we surround ourselves with people filled with negative thoughts and emotions, who aren't mindful in their speech, and whose physical habits are toxic, we're likely to absorb some of these qualities. When we surround ourselves with those who share our aspirations toward greater harmony, greater clarity, purity, and peace, it makes it easier for us to find what we seek.

For example, say I go to a friend's house for a party and everyone present is smoking cigarettes and drinking whiskey and the television is blaring with a very violent movie. To top things off, they are barbecuing burgers and hot dogs on the grill by the pool. Before I know what's happening or can stop my mind from jumping all over the place, I'm going to start to wonder if a cigarette wouldn't feel good, if a shot of whiskey wouldn't make me a little more comfortable. I'll remember how much I used to like burgers, as I watch everyone else enjoying them. The violence on the television screen will surreptitiously pollute my own thoughts so that even after I've left my friend's home, I'll continue to think about the violent images to which I've just been exposed. Suddenly, I have many more internal obstacles to try to transform in order to get back on my own path toward saucha.

As with all practices, we start with awareness, noticing how we feel when we are with certain people and gradually increasing our time with those who nurture and illuminate the Divine presence within. This doesn't mean we have to abandon those close relations who may not be on our exact path, but we need to be thoroughly established in our own practice before we can spend time with certain people without having their energy rub off on us. If children try to climb on a small sapling, they'll break the limbs and it will never grow. But once the sapling has grown into an oak, it can withstand whatever children do to it. We need to be especially protective as we grow into those great oaks. According to the sage Narada, author of the *Bhakti Sutras*:

> Negative companionship should be fully relinquished. . . . Negative companionship is the cause of selfish desire, anger, delusion, forgetting one's spiritual goal, loss of discrimination, and the loss of everything worthwhile. . . . A swelling ocean is raised from the small waves of companionship.[2]

In contrast, it is an invaluable aid to our practice to be surrounded and supported by others who understand and share our aspirations and practices. The venerable Vietnamese Buddhist master Thich Nhat Hanh says:

> The greatest blessing is to have good, wise, kindhearted friends close by. We can't be happy unless we have a sane, healthy space within us and around us. . . . It is a great blessing to be among friends who are practicing. . . . Our community can be a family that sustains us. . . . When we can interact with those who are honorable and have great virtue, we are creating conditions that will bring us lasting

happiness. . . . Creating a nourishing environment is crucial. Only
with this support can we be a source of joy for ourselves and others.[3]

On a more global level, saucha implies doing our part to protect the environment and live in sustainable ways. Some forms of pollution are more obvious than
others, but the more mindful we are the more we can see all the many consequences
that stem from our actions. And the more connected we feel to the environment, the
more likely we are to seek out ways of protecting it.

To begin with, caring for the environment would include things like putting
our trash in the trashcan and doing as much recycling or composting as possible.
Further, the more mindful we are about where our own waste is going, we may find
we can reduce the amount of trash we create to begin with: using fewer bags and less
packaging; and selecting products that can be reused or recycled rather than simply
thrown away to end up in a landfill.

As a society, we are becoming much more conscious of the impact transportation has on the environment. If we are in a position to do it, we can buy cars that are
more fuel-efficient. We can set aside one day a week (or if that's not possible, one day
a month) where we commit to not driving at all. We can use public transportation.
We can bike or walk.

Many of the household and lawn products that we use are toxic not just to our
own health but to the environment as well. When it rains, excess fertilizer runs off
into storm sewers and pollutes streams. Pesticides designed to target certain species
affect entire ecosystems, throwing off the delicate balance of nature. They pose a
demonstrable risk to human health, and they likely bear much responsibility for what
could be the greatest mass extinction event in the planet's history.[4] Amphibians, bats,
and honeybees are dying in huge numbers, and many environmentalists point to
pesticide use as the main culprit.[5] These species are the proverbial canaries in the
coal mine, alerting us to the presence of deadly chemicals that threaten us all. It's not
just a tragedy for the frogs, bats, and bees. A full third of all the food we eat depends
on honeybees for pollination. We need honeybees, and yet we're killing them with

our pesticides. The story of the honeybees is another concrete example of our inter-connectedness, and the dire consequences of our inability to see it.

Much of the environmental damage caused by pesticides comes from agricul-ture, so when we select organic foods over conventional foods we support sustainable and environmentally friendly farming methods. The household use of pesticides is another source of toxicity over which we have complete control.

It is our food choices, however, that have perhaps the biggest personal impact on the environment. We can eliminate not just waste but all the pollution involved in transportation by growing our own food, participating in community gardens and community-supported agriculture (CSAs), and selecting locally produced and organic foods. All of these behaviors are important, but research indicates that the single most impactful personal action we can take to reduce our environmental foot-print is to adopt a plant-based diet.

Cleaning up the environment involves doing our best to refrain from adding our own pollution and doing whatever we can to clean up the mess others may have left. Just as we take care of our own bodies and our homes, we can begin to notice how our actions affect the larger environment and take care of it as our own. If someone throws rotten eggs at my house, I'm going to clean them up, even though I didn't egg my own house. So, too, in addition to not littering ourselves, we might try to compensate for those who do by picking up the plastic bottles we see on the beach or beer cans on the hiking trail. There are many ways we can work at protecting and cleaning up the environment. The point is to begin to see the planet as a part of our own environment and to recognize that taking care of it is a part of our personal practice.

Saucha is also connected to the yama of *brahmacharya*, a teaching that often scares people, as it translates as "celibacy." However, Patanjali is clear that these ethics are for everyone, not just monks, so brahmacharya implies not so much the complete suppression of sexual desire as control of it. It means harnessing our desires and directing that power toward the Divine. A really beautiful expression of this teaching can be seen in the third mindfulness training, as composed by Thich Nhat Hanh. The Five Mindfulness Trainings represent a modernized adaptation of the five precepts of Buddhism, which form the foundation of a basic Buddhist practice. The training reads:

> Aware of the suffering caused by sexual misconduct, I am committed to cultivating responsibility and learning ways to protect the safety and integrity of individuals, couples, families, and society. Knowing that sexual desire is not love, and that sexual activity motivated by craving always harms myself as well as others, I am determined not to engage in sexual relations without true love and a deep, long-term commitment made known to my family and friends. I will do everything in my power to protect children from sexual abuse and to prevent couples and families from being broken by sexual misconduct. Seeing that body and mind are one, I am committed to learning appropriate ways to take care of my sexual energy and cultivating loving kindness, compassion, joy and inclusiveness—which are the four basic elements of true love—for my greater happiness and the greater happiness of others. Practicing true love, we know that we will continue beautifully into the future.[6]

If I'd read this when I was younger I believe I might have avoided causing myself and others much pain. There are so many complex reasons why we engage in sexual relationships. When rooted in deep love and an ability to see the Divine in the other person, these can lead us to happiness and peace. Romantic love can be a glimpse into Divine union, where we feel that the other person moves in our own soul and we in theirs; the boundaries that separate us dissolve and we feel an ecstatic sense of connection. However, we often confuse love with desire, which can lead us and others into great unhappiness. Desire can be very powerful. When we are under its influence we can feel that we've been drugged. We can lose all control, all better judgment. The urge to be with someone, whether we locate that urge in the heart or in the sex organs, can become so strong we are swept away. Blinded by desire, we can't see the full reality or consequences of our actions. Infidelity, unwanted pregnancy, and feelings of remorse and regret are just some of these unwelcome consequences.

Several years ago, under the spell of this kind of deluded desire and really against my own instincts, I entered into a relationship that turned out to be particularly destructive to myself and to others. Once I was out of the relationship I was able to look back with clarity and see how drunk I was with desire and how much it had clouded my judgment. It shook me deeply to recognize how poor my judgment had been. I'd believed the draw I felt was real love, and because I felt the pull located in my heart I hadn't identified it as desire, which is exactly what it was. The most difficult part of the experience was the feeling that I couldn't trust my own judgment. The person with whom I'd been in this relationship turned out not to be the person I thought he was. Though again in retrospect I realized my instincts all along had been warning me to stay away, I hadn't listened.

Shortly after the relationship ended, I happened to encounter a Buddhist monk who'd set up a booth outside one of the local Asian food markets. He was handing out free literature and trying to spread the *Dharma* (the way or great truth of the universe, the core of the Buddha's teachings) to those who wanted to hear it. I was immediately drawn to him and we began talking. He told me it was very important that I be vegetarian. I proudly told him that I wasn't just vegetarian, I was vegan; I even had my own vegan food business. He smiled. "Good, good," he said. And then, "And no sex! No meat and no sex!" I smiled, a bit uncomfortable with the mere mention of the topic. It seemed sort of inappropriate to have a conversation about sex with this middle-aged monk. So I said, "OK, OK," while mentally discarding the last exhortation. He asked if I wanted to be blessed, which of course I did. Then he chanted for a while in a language I didn't understand, touched my head, and gave me the name Wisdom. I left feeling light and happy.

About a week later, I started to think about what the monk had said about no sex. I thought about how bad my judgment had been, how I really didn't trust myself to make decisions about the relationships I was getting involved in. I wasn't ready to become a monastic, but I decided to take a yearlong vow of celibacy. Immediately, I experienced a sense of purity and freedom I can't remember ever having felt before, at least not as an adult. I felt safe and protected. Not long after that, an ex-boyfriend tried to come back into my life. This was someone who'd been very unhealthy for me but whom I still loved deeply. Without that vow, there's a very good chance I would have let this person back into my life and gotten back on the hamster wheel of habitual and destructive patterns that had sabotaged me repeatedly throughout my twenties and thirties. I don't know that I was strong enough on my own to break that cycle. But I used that vow as a shield to give me strength, and I got off the wheel.

About the time that yearlong period was ending, I went on a retreat led by Thich Nhat Hanh. In a beautiful and moving ceremony, I took a vow to observe the Five Mindfulness Trainings, including the third training on true love quoted above. It is not a strict vow of celibacy, but it has had the same protective power for me ever since. When I've felt some desire arising, I've evaluated it in light of the training, and I've made a commitment to honor the vow. This has saved me from making those bad decisions that come from blind desire or loneliness and which so often lead to great unhappiness. When I've felt desire arising, I have looked at where it's coming from and what the consequences would be, and I've worked toward generating real love for all involved. Not through suppression, but through true love, I've watched as the unhealthy desires have dissolved and clear vision has returned. Consequently, I've been able to see the whole truth of the situation clearly enough to make those decisions that lead to true happiness, and to preserve the sense of purity that comes with true love.

The second prong of saucha is purity in speech. Pure speech incorporates the other yogic teachings such as *satya*, or honesty, as well as *ahimsa*, or non-harm. Pure speech is that which reflects our true Divine Self, known as *Atman* to the yogis.

According to the earliest Buddhist scriptures, the historical Buddha taught that right speech had four parts:

1. Abstain from false speech; do not tell lies or deceive.
2. Do not slander others or speak in a way that causes disharmony or enmity.
3. Abstain from rude, impolite, or abusive language.
4. Do not indulge in idle talk or gossip.

Pure speech requires enough awareness for us to pause before we speak and enough discipline to follow these precepts, restraining ourselves from gossip or other malicious discussions. The positive qualities of pure speech are communicating without ego and speaking genuinely and from the heart.

The third prong of saucha, purity of mind, is perhaps the most difficult to practice. We learn to control our actions and even our speech. But how do we control our minds, when thoughts seem to arise on their own volition? We learn in yoga that the key to enlightenment, to happiness, and to peace is to control the mind. Indeed, controlling the mind isn't just a part of yoga. It *is* yoga, as defined by Patanjali. Patanjali's *Yoga Sutras* begins with this definition of yoga: *yoga chitta vritti nirodha*, "Yoga is the control of the mind" (1:2).

What Patanjali means is that we must quiet the competing voices, the cacophonous chatter of the mind, in order to see, hear, and feel the true Self within. Yoga teaches us that the true Self is that pure peace, joy, and compassion we experience when the mind is still and the heart is open enough to dissolve pride and ego.

We look for the small gaps in between the thoughts and allow ourselves to drop into the silence and stillness. In doing so, we discover within ourselves a calm peace and spaciousness. The sages tell us that it is only in this quiet mind that the illusion of separateness dissolves. We are no longer better or worse. We aren't even equal. We are One.

In this still space, free from our limiting ideas about who I think I am and who I think you are, we're able to experience our higher Selves. We connect with the Divine through our daily lives when we see a child walk into traffic and without a second thought (without the obstacle of the mind), and with no concern for our own welfare, we race head-on into traffic to save the child. This is the part of ourselves awakened when we see a woman on the news dying from Ebola, or a child suffering from the effects of chemical warfare in a land on the other side of the world. This is the part of us that bursts through with generosity and compassion when that woman we've been jealous of for years is diagnosed with cancer and we forget all of our animosity and pray for her recovery, not with pity but with real humanity and compassion.

This is the part of us that yoga teaches will outlive these mortal bodies and the ever-changing qualities of ego. The true Self is constant, eternal, forever at peace. We believe we are a wave, with a beginning and an end, separate from all the other waves. Yoga tells us, in truth, that we are the ocean. All of the waves are the ocean. When we discover this eternal, true Self, we realize a harmony within ourselves and come into union with this same divine essence that animates all living beings. This is the true meaning of yoga.

Admittedly, quieting the mind is no easy task. In the *Bhagavad Gita* ("Song of the Lord"), a 700-verse scripture that is widely considered to be the heart of Hinduism and an important scripture for yogis, Lord Krishna, believed by many to be the supreme incarnation of God, counsels a young and confused warrior named Arjuna. From a mystical perspective, Lord Krishna can be seen as representing the ultimate wisdom of the higher Self within each of us. Arjuna can be viewed as the ego-based self with whom we erroneously identify as being our true identity. The *Gita* can be read as a conversation between the Lord and a warrior prince, or as a conversation between the higher Self and the lower self, where we are both Lord Krishna and Arjuna. In this legendary conversation, Lord Krishna tells Arjuna that ultimate peace comes from quieting the mind and controlling the senses. Yet even he admits that, as Arjuna states, "[c]ontrolling the mind is harder than controlling the wind."[7]

This is why Patanjali tells us that peace will only come with consistent, sincere practice, over a long period of time.[8] Taming the mind is a constant practice. In his letter to the Thessalonians in the Christian Bible, the apostle Paul tells us to "pray constantly" (5:17). It's unlikely he intended us to genuflect before an altar around the clock, but rather to regard this whole life as prayer, to look for the Divine in all, gazing always upon the Light within and the Light within others. From a yogic or a Buddhist perspective, prayer is not a supplication to an external being but represents an aspiration, a way to train the mind: to tame it and quiet it.

Traditionally, purity of mind is described as a clear, still lake. The water is so clean and placid that you can see all the way down to the bottom. If we throw rocks into a lake, we cause ripples that obscure the clarity. Our thoughts are like rocks, causing the ripples that cloak our clarity of mind. Any thoughts that create this distortion may be considered impure. So again, the concept of purity here does not carry any particular moral judgment. Those thoughts that lead to clarity and peace of mind are considered pure; those that disturb the mind are considered impure.

Purity of mind comes from being aware of our thoughts and constantly cultivating those thoughts that lead us toward greater peace. When we see that our thoughts are leading us away from peace, we learn to look intently at those thoughts while maintaining our awareness. If we look deeply enough, we can see their origin and begin transforming those habitual thought patterns that lead us away from peace. We learn to see that those thoughts that lead us away from peace are usually coming from the ego. These are the fear-based thoughts—jealousy, resentment, craving, anger—rooted in a feeling of separation, and a corresponding sense of lack and isolation. In a world of separation, we are in constant competition for limited goods. The Eastern traditions can help us see that we are not separate, and that the real treasures (peace and love) are limitless.

As the great Buddhist teacher Shantideva taught, "All the suffering in the world comes from seeking pleasure for oneself. All the happiness in the world comes from seeking pleasure for others."[9] The more we focus on ourselves, the more we reinforce the illusion of separation in which we will never have enough. The more we focus on serving others, the closer we come to the wisdom of interconnection, and the realization that we are not isolated or alone, but are part of the whole—and in that, we are boundless infinite creatures, lacking for nothing.

❀

In yogic and Buddhist philosophy, the senses are often referred to as gates. It's through these gates that we let the world into our own consciousness. So we must guard what comes in through them. The Buddha talked about four kinds of nutriments that come in through the senses and can lead to our happiness or our suffering.[10] The first is the food we eat (discussed below). The second nutriment is sense impressions: what comes into contact with our eyes, ears, nose, tongue, body, and consciousness. When we walk through a shopping mall, we're bombarded with advertisements promoting and watering the seeds of desire within us for material possessions, superficial beauty, wealth, and many other things that lead us away from the fullness of the Divine within. When we watch television or movies, if we don't choose carefully, the programs and films water our own seeds of fear, anger, and ego-based craving and desire.

There is a Buddhist sutra that dramatically illustrates the teaching. The Buddha offered the image of a cow afflicted with a terrible disease that has caused her skin to shed until she has almost none left. Consequently, she is vulnerable to every parasite, insect, and bacterium with which she comes into contact. The Buddha said we are all like this cow, vulnerable to the images we see, the words and conversations we hear or speak, everything we ingest through any of our senses. Our protection, our skin, is our mindfulness. Without mindfulness, all of these impressions invade us and permeate us.[11]

With mindfulness, we can choose what we allow in. When we look at the billboard on the highway advertising a bacon cheeseburger at the next exit, if we are mindful we know the meat itself is toxic to our bodies. We know that many animals suffered to make this one sandwich. We know that the workers in the slaughterhouses have also suffered, and that the environment is being destroyed to produce these burgers. With this level of awareness, we can make the choice not to pull off the freeway but to wait to eat until we can nourish ourselves with pure food. In this way, we nurture our own energy of awareness and compassion, and our understanding of interconnection. In this way, we keep our bodies and our minds pure.

The third nutriment the Buddha spoke of is volition, or will. This is what really drives us. What is the purpose of our life? Are we driven by purely self-serving desires, or are we driven to serve others in some way? If we are driven to be happy, everything we do is fed by that desire. If we are driven to make money, everything we do is directed to that goal. If we are driven to protect living beings, to spread compassion in the world, to promote the healing of the planet, or reconciliation between people, then this is what drives us and this is where we will devote our energy. That which feeds the ego keeps us trapped in a cycle of suffering; that which feeds the Divine within us leads us to happiness and keeps our minds pure and untainted.

The fourth nutriment is consciousness. What seeds in our consciousness do we water? Do we water the seeds of greed, desire, fear, anger, ignorance, or those of compassion, generosity, kindness, respect, and devotion?

In reality, these four nutriments are not separate, but like all the teachings they are interconnected. When we are mindful of one, we take care of the others at the same time. When we are mindful of what we take in through edible food or the sense impressions, we help purify the consciousness. When we generate an energy or volition that is pure, we also purify the consciousness. And when we purify the consciousness, we help ensure that we'll only ingest what is pure in the other three areas as well.

In the *Bhagavad Gita*, Lord Krishna tells us that the way to purity is through devotion. He advises us to make all our actions worship the Divine; to see the Divine within ourselves; to see the Divine within all creation, within all life; and to devote ourselves to that. Again, worship of the Divine here is not worship of an external entity, but of all beings, of the highest good in all beings. Krishna says that when we really see and feel the Divine in all beings, the heart becomes open and is purified. This is the ultimate purity: realizing the true Self and seeing this exists within our own hearts and within all beings. When we're lost in our ego-mind, we're not in our hearts, where we need to be to connect with that Divine presence. In order to let go of ego-based thoughts, we need to feed and nurture ourselves with practices that help us transcend the ego and the idea of a separate self. We practice to quiet the mind and to open the heart.

The deeper truth of yoga is that we're not trying to become pure; we already *are* pure. We've only forgotten this truth; the practices and teachings are there to help us remember. The whole process of purification, the whole path toward enlightenment and wholeness, is not a matter of becoming. It's a matter of realizing, remembering—of letting go of all the layers of forgetting. We are already Divine; we always were pure. We've just gotten lost and are trying to get back home.

Ahimsa (Non-Harm) and a Yogic Diet

> If you want to progress on a spiritual path, you must challenge your actions—including what you eat—as to whether they are authentic expressions of the love and spirit within you. You must ask whether what you are doing bespeaks compassion or indifference to the suffering of others.
>
> As long as you act—and cat—without compassion, you remain mired in the realm of separation, loneliness, and frustration, because you have not yet given voice, with your life, to the great heart within you.—**John Robbins**[12]

In yogic philosophy, the Divine is believed to exist in all living beings, human and nonhuman alike. Based in this understanding, serving God would again not mean serving some external exalted being but each and every being we meet. Krishna tells us that those with true spiritual wisdom "have equal regard for all. They see the same Self in a spiritual aspirant and an outcast, in an elephant, a cow, and a dog" (5:18). Happiness, he says, comes when we see the Divine in all beings, when we worship the Divine "in the hearts of all" (6:30). If the Divine exists in each living being, then our relationship with the Sacred is determined by how we treat all beings. Perhaps this is why ahimsa, or doing no harm to any sentient being, is the first of the yamas of yoga. Ahimsa is the heart and backbone of a yogic practice, or a spiritual practice of any kind.

An essential teaching in all of the Indian spiritual traditions—including Hinduism, Buddhism, Yoga, and Jainism—ahimsa includes not killing any other being, but goes much further. Ahimsa means abstaining from causing any pain or doing any harm to any living being, either by thought, word, or deed. Ahimsa requires us to refrain from harming other humans, the environment, and nonhuman animals, too, by foregoing practices such as meat-eating, hunting, or anything else that causes pain to another living being. Ahimsa implies a release of all enmity and a life lived in harmony with all creatures. More than simply not harming others, ahimsa implies genuine compassion and concern for the welfare of others.

While yoga may be considered a philosophy, it is above all a set of teachings that are meant to be applied and not just talked about or meditated upon. Ahimsa is the most fundamental way we begin to transcend the ego-based illusion of a separate self and in a practical way start to bring ourselves into harmony with all beings. We don't apply ahimsa blindly because someone told us to; spiritual practice must be authentic. Ultimately, we must discover truth for ourselves. The teachings and teachers are there to help us find our way. They help bring the light of awareness to areas that have been hidden in darkness.

As we develop on our spiritual path, our awareness of the world increasingly expands beyond our own self-interest. We become less self-absorbed; we become increasingly aware of how our actions affect others. If we are mindful and looking at our own lives with a genuine intention of applying ahimsa, one of the first areas we will confront is our diet, because for most of us it is the most violent area of our lives. The vow not to kill or harm extends equally to nonhuman animals, and so our habit of eating them is one of the first behaviors we must investigate if we are serious about our practice.

❀

No matter what our spiritual, religious, or metaphysical views, most of us would find our hearts break were we to enter a slaughterhouse. So we look the other way. We close our eyes. We eat with denial. The ancient sages tell us that we find the Divine by looking into "the secret cave of the heart."[13] But if we have to shut our hearts down in order to continue a practice that we sense is not in tune with our hearts, not only do we deny our compassion but we close off the Divine part of ourselves, that Divine core that is the source of all of our own happiness and wisdom.

For the first sixteen years of my life I ate animals without much thought. I don't know that I connected the hamburgers I ate with a being in the world called a cow. I grew up in the suburbs, and so, like many people, the food I ate was completely disconnected from the animals from whom the food came. It didn't occur to me that I was harming anyone. I didn't eat cows; I ate hamburgers. I didn't eat chickens; I ate chicken. I didn't eat pigs; I ate bacon. It was simply not something I questioned. Like everyone else I knew, I'd been doing it as long as I'd been alive. It was as natural as putting one foot in front of the other.

Then I watched a documentary on the meat and dairy industries produced by the animal rights group People for the Ethical Treatment of Animals (PETA). It was absolutely shocking to me. The video consisted of graphic and brutal footage straight from the slaughterhouses. It was simply the truth of what happens behind those closed doors, without a filter.

There's a whole body of work in the world that falls under the heading of BEARING WITNESS. These are straight, objective accounts of tragic events. The idea of this genre is that when truly atrocious events occur, the most authentic, honest, and powerful way to convey the facts is to get out of their way and let them speak for themselves. The myriad undercover factory farm and slaughterhouse documentaries we can now find with a quick Internet search serve this purpose. I became a vegetarian for the first time after seeing this PETA documentary. I say *the first time* because

I'd return to eating animals many times before finally giving up all animal products for good about a decade ago.

By the time I gave up all animal products, I thought I'd expanded my awareness and compassion about as far as possible. I'd come to believe that all those farmed animals deserved to live as much as anyone and that their suffering mattered more than my taste for bacon or cheese, even though I *really* liked bacon and cheese. But I saw my role in their suffering, and I decided I would no longer be a part of it. I believed I was living as peaceful a life as anyone could ask.

Then one day, a cockroach ran across my kitchen floor and instinctively I stomped on him. He didn't die but rather lay on the hardwood floor pitifully flailing his legs and trying to right his half-squished self. This was not a senseless object. This was a creature struggling to live and experiencing some kind of suffering.

The more aware we become, the more we begin to notice all the many ways we harm others. Our understanding of "harm" expands, as does our understanding of "others." As I watched this cockroach struggling on my kitchen floor, I realized for the first time how I'd excluded insects from my circle of compassion, not based on any reasoned principle, but solely on my own lack of awareness and irrational fear.

Despite a lifelong aversion to insects bordering on actual phobia, I decided it was time to stop killing bugs. I realized that my reaction to bugs was very similar to the way some of my friends react (for example) to mice. They find them dirty and grotesque and believe that this justifies their extermination, often in excruciating ways (such as glue traps). I grew up with mice as pets, so I've always thought of them as cute, cuddly, intelligent, and playful, not pests. Seeing the similarity in my own reaction was enough to give me pause. Awareness alone really is a powerful tool of change and growth.

A couple of years ago I was at the sink when I had another one of these sudden flashes of heightened awareness. If you buy organic produce you probably know that it often comes with bugs included. So I wash my kale really well. But one day, as I was standing over the sink, I watched as a tiny grayish mite crawled up a leaf of kale and challenged me to deny his existence. I was paralyzed for a moment. I didn't know whether I should flush him down the drain or smush him with my thumb, or what.

What a mystery all life is, even the smallest life! Yet there's no question that even the tiniest insects are endowed with life and have a will to preserve it. The significance of that is really beyond at least my intellectual capacity to understand. Who am I to play God? So I took the leaf of kale upon which the mite was roaming and laid it outside in the bushes, feeling quite like the Buddha as I liberated him. I was so proud of this Buddha-like respect and compassion and devotion to all life that I think I even noticed goose bumps on my arms as I returned to washing my kale. As I did, I slowly focused in on the tens, probably hundreds, of little mites all being swept down the drain. And all that pride of a moment before went down with them.

The Jains of India adhere to a range of strict practices designed to avoid harming even the simplest life forms. In addition to following a vegetarian diet, they avoid root vegetables such as potatoes, carrots, and turnips in order to protect the tiny creatures who may inhabit the roots. Jain monks and nuns keep muslin cloths over their mouths to prevent inhaling (and thereby harming) flying insects, and they carry small brooms wherever they go so as to gently sweep away any living creatures from their path.

The point is not that we must practice a perfect ahimsa, which in truth is simply impossible, but that we do our best, without allowing the perfect to be the enemy of the good, without giving up because we can't avoid all harm. Our ability to practice ahimsa is largely concurrent with our level of awareness. In order to do no harm, we must see our assumptions and challenge our own beliefs and ideas, as most harm stems either from our ignorance or our bias.

One glaring example of the cruelty that comes from ignorance is slavery. It wasn't that long ago in American history that many white people believed that African Americans were less human than whites and only semi-sentient and thus less capable of suffering. This made it more acceptable to beat them and deprive them of a free life. In fact, enslavement was only possible because of this belief in their inferiority. Enslavement of millions of human beings happened in America because of a false idea rooted in misperception and ignorance.

In the *Diamond Sutra*, the Buddha tells us, "Where there is perception, there is deception."[14] We become what we think, and we create the world we live in from these thoughts. As history teaches us, we must be vigilant in questioning our perceptions. Followers of René Descartes, the French mathematician and father of modern philosophy ("I think, therefore I am"), used to conduct vivisection (live experimentation) on un-anaesthetized dogs and rabbits.[15] They likened their howls and screams to the sounds produced by a church organ when you press one of the keys. In the West today, one would be hard-pressed to find a single scientist with this view. We know dogs are sentient; we know their howls and writhing signal pain.

But what about cows, chicken, fish, or pigs? They scream and writhe, too. Science tells us that the average pig is smarter than the smartest dog. In addition to having complex social interactions and long-term memories, pigs can use reflections in mirrors to find food, operate joysticks with their snouts, and play simple matching games by moving the cursor around a computer screen, showing a capacity similar to primates.[16] According to Donald Broom, Professor of Animal Welfare at University of Cambridge Veterinary School, "[p]igs have the cognitive ability to be quite sophisticated. Even more so than dogs and certainly [more so than] three-year-olds."[17]

Yet, intelligence has never been the best determinant for according compassion. The English utilitarian philosopher Jeremy Bentham said over two hundred years ago:

> The French have already discovered that the blackness of skin is no reason why a human being should be abandoned without redress to the caprice of a tormentor. It may come one day to be recognized, that the number of legs, the villosity of the skin, or the termination of the os sacrum, are reasons equally insufficient for abandoning a sensitive being to the same fate. What else is it that should trace the insuperable line? Is it the faculty of reason, or perhaps, the faculty for discourse? . . . the question is not, Can they reason? nor, Can they talk? but, Can they suffer? Why should the law refuse its protection

to any sensitive being? . . . The time will come when humanity will extend its mantle over everything which breathes. . . .[18]

Even if we don't consider ourselves spiritual, or even if the spiritual tradition with which we identify teaches that animals have no soul, the vast majority of Americans see themselves as animal lovers. Even those of us who don't would almost certainly be disturbed watching a living creature suffer in the way animals raised for agriculture do on a daily basis. The way most of us handle this dilemma is to contract out the raising and killing of animals so we don't have to observe it. By the time the animal flesh or animal secretions arrive on our plates, they're cleaned and dressed with no hint of the actual individual being who not only died for our meal but most likely suffered terribly for the duration of his or her life.

Yoga teaches us not to turn away from what makes us uncomfortable. We learn to become aware of our thoughts and feelings, so we can begin to make choices in our lives that are authentic, that are unified. With practice, we learn to align our thoughts, words, and deeds, and in doing so connect with the Divine Self within, which connects us with the Cosmic Self, the universe, God, Brahma, Buddha (whatever name we use, whatever form we recognize). Yoga teaches us to look for wisdom in our hearts and not our heads, and then to do our best to live in accordance with the Divine wisdom we find there. Yoga's sister science of Ayurveda tells us that if we're not living in accordance with our hearts, we're in real trouble, as that inconsistency will manifest in psychological and physical illness (discussed below).

The Buddha's Take on Non-Harm

Just as ahimsa is the first ethic of yoga, non-killing or ahimsa is also the first precept of Buddhism. As stated in the *Dhammapada*, a collection of the Buddha's own statements, "All beings tremble before danger, all fear death. When a man considers this, he does not kill or cause to kill. All beings fear before danger, life is dear to all. When a man considers this, he does not kill or cause to kill."[19] In his book *The Great Compassion*, Norm Phelps calls this the "classic Buddhist statement of ahimsa," which he defines as not just non-harming but "boundless, universal love and compassion put to work in the world."[20] Cultivating real love for all beings is not only the heart of a Buddhist practice, but the basis of all of our actions in the world, including our thoughts, words, and actions.

Nonetheless, to function in a world of so much suffering, many of us shut down emotionally. We put up armor so we won't have to be hurt. The problem is that it is our very tenderness, our vulnerability itself, that represents our basic seed of goodness and the greatest potential source of joy. The Tibetan Buddhist teacher Chögyam Trungpa Rinpoche likened this to an open wound. It is this raw spot that allows for compassion and for real authenticity. So long as we are wearing armor to protect ourselves, we aren't authentic. So long as we are inauthentic, we remain in a battle with ourselves. We create a sort of schizophrenia within, where our lives and actions in the world aren't in harmony with our hearts. This leads us to live in a state of constant anxiety and fear—primarily a fear of being with ourselves, with our own hearts.

When we stop and look around, we can see that practically our whole society is frantically attempting to ameliorate this anxiety and discomfort through various distractions and escape routes. We can use almost any part of our lives as an escape, as when we seek not just companionship but fulfillment in other people, and thus enter into unhealthy relationships out of the sort of desperation that loneliness creates. We overwork, shop obsessively, eat compulsively, and drink too much. We smoke cigarettes, take drugs, and use sex as an escape from ourselves and from the present moment as it is. But none of these diversions actually rids us of the fear and the sense we can't shake that we are missing something, that we are incomplete. They can certainly offer transient happiness and numb us for a short while. And often, they make us either physically or emotionally sick in the process.

This race never ends. We'll either have to stop running and confront ourselves, or run ourselves to death, literally. The only way to avoid this grueling race is to pause, stay put, and allow ourselves to experience what we've been running from. When we stop, the fear and anxiety melt into tenderness and sadness. We're so afraid of feeling this sadness, but when we do finally experience it we find that the pain of compassion transcends our personal suffering. I've never heard this better expressed than by Chögyam Trungpa Rinpoche:

When you awaken your heart in this way, you find, to your surprise, that your heart is empty. You find that you are looking into outer space. What are you, who are you, where is your heart? If you really look, you won't find anything tangible and solid. Of course, you might find something very solid if you have a grudge against someone or you have fallen possessively in love. But that is not awakened heart. If you search for awakened heart, if you put your hand through your rib cage and feel for it, there is nothing there except for tenderness. You feel sore and soft, and if you open your eyes to the rest of the world, you feel tremendous sadness. This kind of sadness doesn't come from being mistreated. You don't feel sad because someone has insulted you or because you feel impoverished. Rather, this experience of sadness is unconditioned. It occurs because your heart is completely exposed. There is no skin or tissue covering it; it is pure raw meat. Even if a tiny mosquito lands on it, you feel so touched. Your experience is raw and tender and so personal.

The genuine heart of sadness comes from feeling that your nonexistent heart is full. You would like to spill your heart's blood, give your heart to others. For the warrior, this experience of sad and tender heart is what gives birth to fearlessness. Conventionally, being fearless means that you are not afraid or that, if someone hits you, you will hit him back. However, we are not talking about that street-fighter level of fearlessness. Real fearlessness is the product of tenderness. It comes from letting the world tickle your heart, your raw and beautiful heart. You are willing to open up, without resistance or shyness, and face the world. You are willing to share your heart with others.[21]

It's important to note the significant distinction between sadness and depression. Depression comes from focusing on our own stories, our personal dramas and neurosis. Depression represents a disconnection from life, a vacuum, a lack of hope and energy to move with the flow of life. Sadness, in contrast, is the product of tenderness and compassion. It comes when we open ourselves completely to life. It's part of the fullness and abundance of life. Sadness is not without hope, and it can be a strong driving force that propels us directly into the stream of life.

Our aversion to this sadness keeps us from knowing real peace and happiness and being available to help the world. When we allow ourselves to open up to others and feel what is really in our hearts, we'll inevitably touch this deep sadness within. That very tenderness connects us with other beings and fills us with the tremendous love that spills out of our eyes in tears of sorrow and joy. It is our basic goodness and our innate divinity.

The Buddha is said to have experienced his first enlightenment at the age of seven while at a plowing festival with his family. As he sat beneath the bodhi tree, he watched the overburdened animals plowing ceaselessly all day; he saw the plowmen too straining under their work, and he saw all the tiny creatures being killed as the plows dug up the earth. As he watched, he became absorbed in the suffering of all of them, and as he did he lost his sense of self and experienced nirvana for the first time. Rather than being consumed by the suffering he saw, it became a bridge for him. It opened his heart so he was able to connect with all of those beings. As he connected with them and their suffering, he lost the sense of self that keeps us separate from one another. The etymology of the word *compassion* is "to suffer with." In his compassion, he "suffered with" these beings. The separate self dissolved and he found union with all beings. This union is the ultimate fullness, the ultimate joy of enlightenment.

If we live with our eyes and hearts open, we'll certainly be touched by suffering. But the message of the Buddha and of yoga is that this suffering is not personal, and it isn't depressing. It's not the suffering that makes our lives unbearable; in fact, it's the opposite. It's a suffering that makes real joy possible, the joy that comes with our ability to give, love, and help, to serve and to be useful. In opening our hearts to others and living a life rooted in ahimsa we begin to live in harmony with our Divine nature, with our own hearts. We begin to live in harmony and union with each other, and our lives become richer, fuller, and more meaningful.

Satya—Truthfulness

In the twelve-step program of Alcoholics Anonymous, there's a fundamental conviction that for the program to work and for a person to recover from the deadly disease of alcoholism, one thing is absolutely necessary: one must be "rigorously honest" with oneself. In fact, it's a basic premise of the program that those who are this honest with themselves will succeed. But the elders of the program also recognized there was little hope for those few unfortunate souls who were "constitutionally incapable" of such honesty, conceding that "their chances are less than average."[22] The same could be said for those of us attempting to walk a spiritual path, or seeking health and wellness, peace and happiness. If we truly desire good health, happiness, authenticity, and freedom, we must be rigorously honest with ourselves. Anything else is a setup for failure.

Satya, or honesty, is the second of Patanjali's ethics, which are meant to be universal in application. Honesty is not just for monks. No matter what our status in life, Patanjali says we must be truthful in order to achieve happiness. The virtue of honesty is second only to ahimsa in yogic philosophy. Satya implies honesty in both word and thought. Inner peace, upon which all other peace depends, is only possible when we are honest with ourselves and others.

Honesty in Thought

Dishonesty in thought, otherwise known as denial or suppression, is perhaps the most damaging form of dishonesty. When we try to hide from ourselves we become disconnected from the only true source of joy and peace available to us, our own hearts. Denial leaves us with a sense of discomfort, a nagging feeling just over our shoulder that causes us to doubt ourselves in almost everything we do. This doubt becomes generalized anxiety and insecurity. If we cannot trust ourselves, how could we trust anything or anyone?

Denial as a method of manipulating ourselves only works if we can successfully block our inner voice, our innate wisdom. This takes some effort. As a society, we've gotten quite good at it. In order to mute our own hearts, we turn up the radio, flip on the TV, call a friend (any friend will do), search the Internet, eat, drink, shop, gamble, take drugs, cling to relationships, and do almost anything else to avoid the silence, in which the whispers of truth cannot be ignored.

From a yogic perspective, this is an inevitable prescription for suffering. Yoga teaches us that the root cause of all our suffering is a fundamental disconnection from the Divine Self. Only by returning to the Divine within can we find peace. But if the truth is within and we are trying to avoid it, we have to constantly run from ourselves in order to avoid the truth that scares us.

Sometimes it's inconvenient to confront the truth. Sometimes when we do confront it we become uncomfortable with our current choices and the only way to ease the discomfort is to make changes we don't want to make. It is attachment to our habits and our beliefs that hinders us most on our path toward the Light.

As we become more aware, we discover that no matter what truth we've been running from, we only find peace by looking it squarely in the eye and accepting it. Once we stop running from the great wave that's been rising within us and allow it to wash over us completely, we are released from fear. There's nothing to run from anymore. Fear is replaced by a calm and gentle acceptance of what is true. This direct engagement with reality liberates us from fear and brings us back to life.

Honesty in Speech

The second component of satya is honesty in our speech. This has to do with how we communicate with others. In part, speaking the truth means speaking our own truths, expressing what is important to us, rather than bottling up or stifling our feelings and emotions. We do this for so many reasons. Sometimes we stay quiet to protect others; sometimes we fear others' reactions. It is primarily fear that prevents us from being honest. By the same logic, as Sri Swami Satchidananda taught, "[w]ith establishment in honesty, the state of fearlessness comes."[23] When we know we're always going to be honest, we have nothing more to hide. We are freed from our anxieties. We can stop hiding and come out into the open where we can stand up tall and breathe.

Satya doesn't mean that we have to be or should be callous or hurtful about expressing that truth. We don't practice any one principle in isolation. In order to practice satya in conjunction with the other yamas, or ethical principles, such as ahimsa, we want to strive to express our truths with gentleness and sensitivity. We want to make a sincere effort to communicate in a way that promotes understanding and peace. As the Vedic maxim counsels, *Satyam bruyat priyam bruyat*, "Speak what is truthful, speak what is pleasant."

When interpreting and trying to live by any doctrine, we must seek to understand not just the letter but the spirit of that doctrine. More than simply not telling lies, satya implies educating ourselves about the world in which we live, at least enough so we can skillfully avoid doing harm. Willful blindness is just another form of denial and self-deception. We cannot avoid harming until we first become willing to honestly look at how we may be causing others harm.

Of course, we know our food choices have a major impact on our own bodies, but they also deeply affect other living beings, human and nonhuman, as well as the planet. It's a difficult realization for most of us to come to that, despite the great compassion we have in our hearts, we may find ourselves entrenched in certain practices that harm others. I personally resisted this idea for about two decades before I was able to believe the information in front of me. I didn't want to see how harmful my actions were because I wasn't ready to change, and I wasn't ready to accept the world as it is. But as the ancient Chinese proverb goes, "To close one's eyes does not ease another's pain." To be honest is to live with our eyes open. Only when we do so is there a chance that we can use our lives in a way that can ease the other's pain, which is key to realizing our own happiness and well-being.

Asteya and *Aparigraha* (Non-Stealing and Non-Greed)

The third and fifth of Patanjali's yamas, *asteya* (non-stealing) and *aparigraha* (non-greed), are closely related. We steal because of greed. We steal because we desire what isn't ours. We desire things that we believe will bring us happiness. In the culture we live in, more is better. Bigger is better. But bigger cars, bigger steaks, bigger houses are destroying us and our planet.

In this world, we're constantly being told that we'd be happier if we consumed and possessed more stuff. We're all searching for happiness, and those pretty people in the advertisements look so happy. Patanjali would say that possessing and consuming aren't steps on the path to peace. Trying to find happiness in the plasma TV we can't afford, or the fancy speedboat the neighbors just acquired, or the silky hair in the shampoo commercial, is like the man who searches all over the house for the glasses that are on top of his head. We're looking in the wrong places for something we've had all along.

One of my favorite Vedic stories is about the small musk deer who live high in the Himalayas. Every spring, they detect a fragrance in the air—something like the scent of jasmine or lilacs we smell in the early spring. The odor is so sweet and enticing that the deer begin running with increasing desperation through the forest in search of its origin. They go mad in their search, which ends tragically as they ram into trees and leap off the mountain peaks and crash to their deaths: all for an aroma they never realize is produced by a gland in their own bodies. So too, what we seek is within.

Asteya includes the obvious prohibitions such as "Don't rob a bank," or "Don't take your senile grandmother's jewels," and maybe we see the reasoning here. But upon reflection, we might realize that we take what isn't ours in subtler ways. Just as when we tried to understand the true meaning of ahimsa, we can expand our understanding of asteya to include more ways of taking what isn't ours and a broader understanding of who the "other" is. Besides outright stealing, maybe we maintain some relationships in our lives because we think we have something to gain from them; or perhaps we take advantage of the generosity of our families or friends. If we pause to evaluate our relationship with nonhuman animals and the environment honestly, we might realize we're in almost constant violation of this principle.

Animal agriculture is a system that could not survive otherwise. It's based on the institutionalized practice of stealing babies from their mothers, using other creatures' bodies to produce products that we consume, and ultimately taking their very lives for our own sensory pleasure. We take and take and take from the animals, and when we pause to consider what it is we give them in return (food, water, shelter, life itself), we can see that even these are given out of self-interest.

The same is often true regarding our relationship with the Earth. As a society, we've been exploiting the land for centuries. Gandhi said, "There is enough in this world for every man's need but not for his greed."[24] We live in a time when we can witness the stark truth of these words. We're at a tipping point, where we're taking more than the world can provide.

The only way to understand this self-sabotaging behavior is in our mistaken idea that happiness will come from our possessions, from the things we consume. We don't see that we steal from ourselves. The more we can amass, we think, the happier we'll be. Actually, according to Patanjali, the Buddha, and most other spiritual traditions, the exact opposite is true. We must let go of our attachments to possessions in order to find real happiness. Yoga teaches us that we'll find happiness when we learn to stop taking what doesn't belong to us, to live in a way that makes life possible for all, and to look into our hearts for real fullness and abundance.

Yogic Ethics and Animal Welfare

Yoga is a system for developing inner peace, finding happiness and union with our true selves, and living in harmony with ourselves and the world. And it works, if we practice and apply the teachings to our actual lives. How we treat others is not only of central importance to our own spiritual practice, it *is* our spiritual practice. In this respect, the way we as a society treat animals is an area that needs a major overhaul, beginning with simply including them as relevant beings in the moral equation.

We exploit animals in just about every way imaginable, from using their carcasses and pelts to decorate our bodies with fur-trimmed coats, leather jackets, and feather earrings, to using their bodies to test the efficacy of our medicines and cosmetics. We tear them away from their families and imprison them in small cages so we can enjoy a family day at the zoo, the circus, or the aquarium, never considering that like us they desire freedom, have their own interests, and experience a full range of complex psychological and emotional states. All of these relationships need to be re-evaluated in the light of ahimsa, asteya, aparigraha, and the other essential values of the spiritual path, such as compassion and selflessness. But it is our food choices that have the largest impact on the nonhuman animals, at least in terms of numbers:

> Today's concentrated animal production systems are dedicated to producing meat as cheaply as possible while achieving certain standards of taste, texture, and efficiency. Confinement systems are designed to produce animals of marketable weight in less time. . . . [A]nimals are kept in more crowded conditions, are subject to a number of chronic and production-related diseases, and are unable to exhibit natural behaviors. In addition, the animals are often physically altered or restrained.[25]

When confronted with the reality of animal suffering, most people will say something like "I just don't want to know," or "It's too terrible, I can't even think about it." I know because this was my own reaction for many years. Denial and suppression about how we feel about the animals we eat are so pervasive they're as much of a cultural blind spot as a personal one. The most destructive part of denial is that the very feelings we suppress are crucial for us to tap into in order to live truly loving, happy lives, or to create a loving, peaceful world. Unpleasant as it is to consider, we must see the truth and be honest about what we see. Only then can we make choices that manifest the truths of our Divine hearts.

More than nine billion animals are raised and killed annually for food in the United States alone, and that number does not include fish.[26] In the U.S., we eat more than a million animals an hour: a figure so stunning I think I've redone the math about twelve times to see if I was correct. Unbelievable as it sounds, there are no federal laws governing the conditions under which any of these animals are raised.[27] Animals are increasingly raised in massive indoor structures housing thousands of cows, chickens, and pigs. These are known as factory farms or concentrated animal feeding operations (CAFOs), and they account for ninety-nine percent of all animal products on the market.[28]

Animals raised on factory farms aren't able to exhibit natural behaviors. They spend their lives in dark, overcrowded warehouses subjected to a range of standard industry practices that would lead to criminal charges in all fifty states if they were done on dogs or cats. But farmed animals are excluded from animal-cruelty statutes in almost every state. The only laws protecting them are the Twenty-Eight Hour Law, which applies to transit, and the Humane Slaughter Act, both of which offer only nominal protections.[29]

The Twenty-Eight Hour Law provides that when animals are being transported for slaughter, the vehicle must stop every twenty-eight hours and the animals must be let out for exercise, food, and water. Many truck drivers do not adhere to this rule; the law is rarely, if ever, enforced, and it does not apply to birds.[30] Furthermore, during those twenty-eight hours, animals are routinely crowded in trucks with no food, water, or protection against weather extremes.[31] Many die in transit; many more arrive at the slaughterhouse too sick and injured to walk. These animals are called "downers" and are dragged with chains to the killing floor. Downers are often dairy cows who begin their long journeys to slaughter already in a weakened condition.[32]

The Humane Slaughter Act is similarly limited. It requires only that livestock be stunned prior to slaughter. Many recent undercover investigations show that animals routinely go to slaughter without being rendered unconscious by the stun.[33] Even the government concedes that many plants fail to stun the animals properly prior to slaughter and that government enforcement of the act is weak.[34] Birds, who make up ninety percent of all animals slaughtered in the United States, are entirely exempt from the act. The act also excludes rabbits, fish, and other animals routinely raised for human consumption.

Eggs

Around ninety-five percent of commercially available eggs come from egg factories, where the birds are held in fourteen-inch wire "battery cages," each holding five to eight birds. The animals are packed in so tightly they aren't even able to spread their wings. They spend their whole lives in conditions that can only produce constant physical and psychological distress. To prevent aggression due to the stress of such unnatural living conditions, chicks are debeaked, which is a euphemistic way of saying a part of their beaks is seared off without any anesthesia. The cages extend from one end of the barn to the other and are stacked on top of one another so the birds on all but the top row are constantly showered with the urine and feces of other birds.[35] The wire on which the birds stand bites into their feet, causing them to develop painful and often infected sores, which often kill them.[36] Furthermore, their wings are routinely caught in the wire.

After two years, the hens' bodies are spent and their production declines. No longer useful to the industry, they are sent to slaughter, where because birds are exempt from the Humane Slaughter Act, they are not required to be rendered unconscious before they are shackled, dragged through an electrocution bath, have their throats slit, and are then dropped into boiling water. By the time they arrive at the slaughterhouse, one study has shown, approximately twenty-nine percent of the hens already have broken bones caused by lack of exercise, calcium depletion, and rough handling.[37] According to the United States Department of Agriculture (USDA), an estimated one million chickens and turkeys are boiled alive each year in U.S. slaughterhouses, because the speed of the kill line (the faster the kill line, the higher the profits) makes it impossible for workers to ensure that the birds are dead before they are dropped into the scalding water.[38] They endure all of this without pain medicine.

To boost egg production on the modern farm, hens often undergo a process known as forced molting. Molting refers to the process whereby a hen loses all of her feathers and grows new ones. In nature this happens once a year usually during the fall so the hen will have full new plumage to keep her warm through the winter. While she's molting, she stops laying eggs as her body directs most of its energy to growing the new feathers. On factory farms, hens are manipulated into molting on a planned schedule that increases profit. Forced molting means the molt will be shorter and the hens will continue to lay eggs when market egg prices are highest. This is achieved through starvation. Typical starvation periods are between five and fourteen days. The USDA estimates there are over six million hens in the United States who are being systematically starved in their cages at any given time.[39] All of these conditions make the life of an egg-laying hen one of the most stressful and miserable of all farmed animals.

Perhaps the dirtiest secret of the egg industry is what happens to the male chicks at the hatchery. Egg-laying hens can only survive for a year or two because the process of industrialized egg laying is so devastating to their bodies. After a year, most hens can no longer walk. Many die in their cages, and others are no longer able to produce eggs at a profitable rate so are sent to slaughter. Accordingly, there is a high turnover rate among laying hens, and in order to replenish the flock, other hens are constantly bred at hatcheries. For every female chick born, a male hatches as well. He has no value to the egg-laying industry, and is a different breed than those used for meat, so he has no commercial worth either. The result is that about two hundred million male chicks are killed annually. It makes no difference whether these chicks are ultimately destined for the battery cages or an organic cage-free or free-range farm: male chicks are useless to any commercial operation. The most common methods of killing them are gassing and maceration.[40]

Chickens

Broiler chickens are selectively bred and genetically altered to produce bigger thighs and breasts, the parts most in demand. This breeding creates birds so heavy that their bones cannot support their weight. As a result, they can hardly stand let alone move around without constant pain. Many end up spending their lives lying in their own waste, developing open wounds that are prone to infection.[41] Chickens bred to be eaten are raised in overcrowded houses with as many as twenty thousand birds in one shed, providing less than one square foot of space for each animal.[42] Their beaks and toes are severed without anesthesia, and the broiler houses are usually kept darkened at all hours so the animals eat as many hours in the day as possible. As they are bred to grow fast they reach market weight and are sent to slaughter when they are only seven weeks old. Americans kill and eat more chickens than any other farmed animal. Nearly nine billion of them are killed every year in the United States alone. The lives they lead before slaughter involve such extreme suffering that hundreds of millions of them die before they even make it to the slaughterhouse.[43]

In order to treat any living being in this way, we must create a belief that chickens are somehow oblivious to their surroundings, to pain, and to the conditions of their lives. But that is not what science or our own instincts tell us if we spend any time in the presence of any bird. According to one psychologist and animal behaviorist,

> If, as the evidence indicates, animals are aware, and birds have human-like intelligence, emotions, and personalities, then . . . modern humans have been fundamentally wrong about the nature of basic reality. Since they have been mistaken about their closest and most common wild neighbors, the birds, they need to reassess and reevaluate their presumed understanding of reality and their relationship to everything around them, beginning with birds and extending out to all animals and all of nature.[44]

Pigs

Pigs are considered one of the smartest species on the planet, along with chimpanzees and dolphins.[45] Standard farming practice is to remove piglets from their mothers when they are less than one month old. The piglets' tails are severed, their teeth cut, and the males castrated—all without any pain relief. Anyone who did these things to a dog would be sent to jail. Yet because of some artificial distinctions we've drawn, we make dogs our companions and pigs our food.[46]

Pigs spend their entire lives in overcrowded pens on a tiny slab of concrete. More than 170,000 die in transport each year, and over 420,000 are crippled by the time they arrive at the slaughterhouse.[47] Breeding sows live in tiny metal cages called gestation crates where they cannot so much as turn around. Shortly after giving birth, they are again forcibly impregnated. This cycle continues for years until their bodies finally give up and they are sent to slaughter.

Beef Cows

Driving through the countryside we may see cows destined to become beef happily grazing in pastures. This is the picture of farming most of us quite naturally have in our minds since we don't routinely see the inside of a slaughterhouse or a factory farm. These places are, for obvious reasons, intentionally kept hidden. Instead, we see bucolic scenes where herds of cattle, babies with their mothers, graze languidly amidst tall grasses and fields dotted with romantic old barns and grain silos. Looking at such scenes, it's easy to tell ourselves stories like "The animal lived a good life until he was slaughtered."

The truth is that most beef cattle will spend the first six months of life with their mothers grazing in this idyllic way, except for the pain of having hot iron seared into their flesh when they're branded in order to identify them as property. Then everything changes. The calf is forcibly weaned from his mother and moved into a pen, where he'll begin to eat from a trough and be introduced to corn so he can put on weight in an unnaturally short period of time.[48]

Cows are ruminants, which means they have four compartments to their stomach, including the rumen. A ruminant digests plant-based food by initially softening it through bacterial compounds within the first compartment of the stomach, then regurgitating the semi-digested mass, known as cud, and chewing it again. This process of chewing the cud to break it down further and stimulate digestion is called "ruminating." But the rumen is evolved to deal with grass, not corn, which is very starchy and too difficult to digest. Because they can't properly digest the corn, gas builds up and can't escape. The rumen expands like a balloon, putting pressure on the internal organs, which will ultimately kill the animal if not treated.[49]

As soon as the cow is switched to corn, he develops digestive problems. He gets bloat and stops ruminating. Corn-fed cows are also susceptible to acidosis, which eventually leads to ulceration of the rumen. Bacteria escape from the rumen into the bloodstream and end up in the liver, creating abscesses. According to bestselling author Michael Pollan, fifteen to thirty percent of all cow livers are too abscessed for people to eat. But overall, it's still more profitable to fatten cows up on corn, so the diseased liver is seen as acceptable collateral damage.[50]

Not long ago, cows were slaughtered at the age of four or five, but it's much more profitable to fatten them up faster and kill them sooner. This accelerated weight gain is only accomplished by a diet of corn, protein, and fat supplements. But feeding them this diet will kill them before they ever get to market unless they're treated prophylactically with antibiotics, which explains why ninety-five percent of the antibiotics used worldwide are given to farmed animals who aren't sick but who'd likely die from illness and disease if they weren't given them.[51]

By the age of about eight months, all beef cows are sent to the feedlot, where they continue eating corn and are crowded by the thousands into long, dusty, open-air pens with no protection from the elements. They stand ankle deep in their own manure, inhaling toxic, bacteria-filled air. They will live here until the age of about fourteen months, at which point they will be trucked to slaughter.[52]

Dairy

It's easy to see how eating meat harms animals, but many people struggle to understand how dairy could cause any harm. The truth is that the dairy industry leads just as inevitably to death as the meat industry does, and often with more suffering for the animals before they get there.

In the beginning of the twentieth century, average annual milk production for a Holstein cow was seven thousand pounds. Today the average dairy cow is forced to produce nineteen thousand pounds a year. While the natural lifespan of a cow is twenty-five years, a dairy cow is usually slaughtered between three and five years, by which point her body is destroyed and she can hardly stand due to calcium depletion. It's estimated that forty percent of dairy cows are lame by slaughter.[53]

As dairy cows only produce milk for about ten months after giving birth, once a year or so they are forcibly impregnated on a machine the industry calls the "rape rack." Female calves are kept to replenish the herd and male calves are usually sent to veal crates. When dairy cows become unable to produce adequate amounts of milk they are sent to slaughter and turned into low-quality ground beef.[54]

Veal calves are kept in small wooden crates that prevent movement and inhibit muscle growth so the meat will be tender. They are fed an iron-deficient diet that makes them anemic and keeps their flesh pale, which, for some reason, is considered desirable for the consumer. Veal calves spend their short four months of life in intensive confinement, alone and deprived of light. Veal calves are a "by-product" of the dairy industry. The USDA explains that "[v]eal is the meat from a calf or young beef animal. A veal calf is raised until about 16 to 18 weeks of age, weighing up to 450 pounds. Male dairy calves are used in the veal industry. Dairy cows must give birth to continue producing milk, but male dairy calves are of little or no value to the dairy farmer. A small percentage are raised to maturity and used for breeding."[55] Contrary to popular belief, whether our dairy comes from a conventional farm or an organic or "humane" farm, all of the above practices are standard across the industry, a fact that should make us question just what the label "humane" means on a carton or a meat or dairy product.

Fish

For every cow we consume, we eat fourteen hundred fish,[56] which makes it particularly poignant that we too readily discount the misery that these sea creatures endure. In the United States, as in most countries, no laws protect fish from inhumane treatment. Even those of us who are naturally sensitive to the suffering of mammals often find more difficulty empathizing with fish. Many of us don't even think of fish as animals. It comes as a surprise to many that the pain receptors in fish are similar to those of mammals. Researchers have concluded that "fish have the capacity for pain perception and suffering."[57] When fish are pulled from the water, they begin to suffocate. Their gills often collapse and their swim bladders can rupture because of the sudden change in pressure. Fish are most often killed by being repeatedly hit on the head, bleeding out, suffocating, or freezing. If you've ever stepped on a fishhook and experienced shooting pain drive deep into your flesh, then you can begin to understand how a fish feels when she is hooked by a fishing line. Our pain receptors are similar, so we experience pain similarly.

Beyond their capacity for physical suffering, fish lead much richer and more complicated lives than many of us would imagine. According to world-renowned animal behaviorist Dr. Jonathan Balcombe, "fish representatives recognize individual 'shoal mates,' acknowledge social prestige, track relationships, eavesdrop on others, use tools, build complex nests, and exhibit long-term memories."[58]

According to the Animal Welfare Institute, about half of the fish consumed globally are farmed as opposed to wild caught.[59] Like the land-based factory farms, fish farms are often characterized by overcrowding, disease, and pollution caused by high concentrations of excrement and uneaten food. As many as one third of farmed fish experience a slow and painful death caused by disease and parasites. As Nick Cooney tells us in his revelatory book *Veganomics*, "[s]ome have their face or flesh chewed off by sea lice."[60] Pollution and disease also pose a threat to wild species, as do the hundreds of thousands of fish who escape farms and threaten the genetic diversity and survival of native species.[61]

For health and even environmental reasons, we are often urged to give up red meat and pig products. This advice, combined with our natural instinct to connect more with pigs and cows than we do with chicken and fish, lead many of us to switch from red meat and pork to eating more chicken and fish. However, when we consider the research, we see that farmed fish likely endure more suffering than any other animal, followed closely by chickens and egg-laying hens. Therefore, if we are interested in reducing as much suffering as possible, the first, rather than the last, animal products we should give up are fish, chicken, and eggs.[62]

The Environment

Livestock production is one of the major causes of the world's most pressing environmental problems including global warming, land degradation, air and water pollution, and loss of biodiversity.—**Food and Agriculture Organization of the United Nations**[63]

According to all the major nongovernmental environmental groups and international scientific bodies, climate change is the single greatest threat to the environment and humanity of our time. There's no question that Earth's temperature is rising. According to NASA, our current rate of warming has not been seen in the past thirteen hundred years, and Earth's average surface temperatures could rise between two and six degrees Celsius by the end of the twenty-first century. While Earth has experienced several cycles of warming and cooling in its long history, scientists agree the current warming trend is not part of a natural cycle.[64]

Climate change is caused by human activity. Climate scientists, including those from the U.S. Environmental Protection Agency (EPA), tell us that if we don't reverse global warming now, we're facing a host of calamitous consequences related to weather patterns, health, wildlife, melting glaciers, and rising sea levels. The increase in Earth's temperature has already begun to lead to coastal flooding, more extreme weather, the spread of disease, and mass extinctions. Global warming is caused by greenhouse gas (GHG) emissions. The most destructive of these is methane, and the number-one producer of methane is livestock.

The livestock sector generates considerable GHG emissions.[65] This is due to a combination of factors including the carbon dioxide (CO_2) emitted in the transport of animals, deforestation related to cattle grazing, and cultivation of feed crops. Even more significant is the methane itself, a greenhouse gas that is twenty-one times more powerful than CO_2. A conservative estimate by the United Nations calculates that animal agriculture is responsible for 14.5 percent of GHG emissions.[66] A 2009 study by Robert Goodland and Jeff Anhang, titled "Livestock and Climate Change: What If the Key Actors in Climate Change Are . . . Cows, Pigs, and Chickens?" placed animal agriculture's contribution of GHGs at a whopping fifty-one percent of annual worldwide emissions.[67] Based on either statistic, it is now clear that animal agriculture is a significant contributor to global warming.[68]

The environmental problems associated with animal agriculture aren't limited to climate change. Increased consumption of animal products means more use of limited resources such as water and land, as well as more fertilizers, pesticides, fuel, and polluting waste. According to the Worldwatch Institute, "The human appetite for animal flesh is a driving force behind virtually every major category of environmental damage now threatening the human future—deforestation, erosion, fresh water scarcity, air and water pollution, climate change, biodiversity loss, social injustice, the destabilization of communities, and the spread of disease."[69]

Next to climate change, fresh water is probably the most pressing environmental problem we face today. Worldwide, 3.4 million people die each year from water-related disease, and 780 million people are without access to clean drinking water.[70] Freshwater makes up only 2.5 percent of all water on Earth. With our current global population, it's essential that water be properly managed, distributed, and protected. The United Nations estimates that by 2025 a full 1.8 billion people will be without access to fresh drinking water as a result of climate change, population growth, and poor water management. Given these facts, it's nothing less than obscene that we use 630 gallons of water to produce a single hamburger.[71]

A study conducted by researchers at Loma Linda University found that animal-based diets use almost three times more water, two-and-a-half times more raw energy, and thirteen times more polluting chemical fertilizers than do plant-based diets.[72] Just growing feed crops for livestock consumes fifty-six percent of the water in the United States.[73]

The environmental issues raised by agriculture are inextricably connected to world hunger. Twenty million people worldwide die as a result of malnutrition, and one billion people will suffer from malnourishment and food insecurity.[74] The World Health Organization says that malnutrition is a factor in at least half of the twelve million childhood deaths that occur each year. In theory, we can feed about nine billion people worldwide—but not when half the world's crops and at least a third of the world's fish catch feed livestock. For example, in the United States, five percent of the oats grown are for human consumption; the other ninety-five percent go to feed livestock. This represents tremendous inefficiency when humans could eat those crops directly.[75]

Animal-based foods (such as meat, dairy, and eggs) are highly resource-intensive and therefore unsustainable given the world population of seven billion and counting. It takes thirteen times more water and eighteen times more land to feed a meat eater than to feed a vegan. Forty thousand pounds of potatoes can be grown on one acre of land, whereas only two hundred and fifty pounds of beef can be produced on that same acreage. An acre of cereal can provide five times more protein than an acre of beef, and an acre of legumes such as lentils, beans, and peas can produce ten times as much protein. The estimated percentage of protein wasted by cycling grain through livestock is a shocking ninety percent.[76]

Forty-five percent of the planet is already being used to raise livestock.[77] With per-capita meat consumption rising along with population and economic growth, overall meat consumption has already increased fivefold in the past fifty years and is expected to double from current levels by 2050.[78] Whether this means an increase in factory farms and a doubling of all of the pollution and suffering associated with them, or doubling the amount of land for agriculture, it's hard to imagine how such an increase could be possible let alone sustainable.

Animal agriculture is also a major driver of deforestation as trees are cut to create more grazing land. This has been especially true in Latin America, where seventy to eighty percent of the Amazon rainforest has been destroyed for cattle grazing or to raise crops for animal feed.[79] The cattle are responsible for major land degradation due to erosion and overgrazing.[80]

The Brazilian Amazon has been hit particularly hard, where ninety percent of its deforestation is due to cattle grazing or cultivating soybeans to feed cattle. Indeed, I witnessed this destruction firsthand. Brazil is a massive country, so we had to drive great distances in between the different regions we visited. En route, we passed through a seemingly endless expanse of flat and barren pasture, all of it formerly rainforest, now grazing land for the eight million cows who are exploited annually in Brazil for their flesh or for dairy.

Our first destination was a private preserve covered by primary and lush rain-forests and home to a wide array of species, many of which are endangered, such as the jaguar, bush dog, puma, giant anteater, sloth, and several primates—including one endangered white-whiskered spider monkey who stuck his tongue out at me right before urinating on my head (for me, a clear highlight of the trip!). In order to access the preserve, we drove past hundreds of acres of ranches and then had to travel through another cattle ranch, where a menacing-looking cowboy with a cigarette dangling from his lip let us in through a gate and waved us through to use the private road that led to the boat launch at the river. On one side of the river, the forest was gone, likely through the slash-and-burn techniques used to clear most forests in Latin America. On the other side was dense primary rainforest, with the river serving as a demilitarized zone between them. The cattle ranchers had stripped everything up to the river; it was only because of the preserve's private owner that the rainforest on the other side of the river had been protected.

Though some statutes are now in place to protect local wildlife, ranchers continue to kill the animals who come out of the forest to hunt their cattle, including many of the big cats. But the ranchers are also realizing that tourism dollars are to be had in protecting these animals, whom ecotourists like us will pay to see in the wild. This has led to a strange and one might even say twisted marriage of cattle ranching and ecotourism.

One "eco-lodge" we stayed at illustrated this incongruous model. We'd drive the dusty road through the owner's cattle ranch on the way to the protected forest where we'd all admire the wild animals. Along the way, we'd see mother cows nestling their newborn calves or sows with their piglets running behind them trying to find a nipple to suckle. I asked to stop the truck once to visit with the pigs. One of the other tourists on the safari truck, a friendly Dutchman, called out, "We don't stop for domestic pigs!" Everyone laughed and the truck bumped along until we screeched to a halt at the next sighting of a "wild" animal.

One night at dinner, the owner came out to talk to the guests. He spoke inspiringly about the importance of conservation and how much he and others in the Brazilian ecotourism movement had accomplished. When I asked him about the direct conflict between cattle ranching and preservation, he recoiled a bit and after a pause responded, "I'm an environmentalist. I don't deal with food." Maybe one day he'll come to realize, as former cattle rancher turned animal rights activist Howard Lyman says in the documentary *Cowspiracy*, "You can't be an environmentalist and eat animal products. Period."[81] And if that's true, you certainly can't be an environmentalist and raise animals for food.

Yet another environmental issue related to animal agriculture is the mass quantities of waste produced when large quantities of animals are housed in factory farms. With the global shift away from small farms toward larger corporate entities, the problem has intensified so drastically that some operations produce as much waste as an entire city.[82] Traditionally, waste produced by livestock would naturally fertilize the land, but by concentrating thousands of animals in indoor buildings, the modern factory farm has become almost entirely disconnected from the land and has nowhere to return such mass quantities of ordure. The result is what the industry calls "lagoons," which is an apt term for an industry shrouded in euphemism and Orwellian doublespeak. The lagoons are massive cesspools often the size of several football fields that are found near every major factory farm in America.

These lagoons sometimes burst or their contents are intentionally spread on nearby cropland without being treated. Runoff after rains or rupture contaminates local waterways, causing serious damage to the environment, local wildlife, and human populations as well. Waste runoff from chicken and pig factory farms in Maryland and North Carolina is believed to have contributed to outbreaks of *Pfiesteria piscicida*, a complex flagellate organism that killed millions of fish and caused skin irritation, short-term memory loss, and other cognitive problems in humans.[83] Residents who live near CAFOs frequently report irritation to their eyes, noses, and throats, along with a decline in the quality of life and increased incidents of depression, tension, anger, confusion, and fatigue.[84] Furthermore, factory farms are most often located in communities of color and poverty, making this an issue of concern for anyone interested in environmental justice or environmental racism.

Nutrients in animal waste also cause algal blooms, which consume oxygen in water, leading to "dead zones" that support no aquatic life. A dead zone in the Gulf of Mexico fluctuates in size each year, extending to 8,500 square miles in the summer of 2002 and over 7,700 square miles in the summer of 2010.[85] Lagoons also release ammonia, a toxic form of nitrogen that also causes algal blooms that kill fish.

Our insatiable appetite for animal flesh and animal by-products is also one of the leading causes of loss of biodiversity globally. Overconsumption has depleted all seventeen of the world's major fishing areas, which have reached or exceeded their natural limits. At least one third of all global fish catch is fed to livestock, and many scientists predict the total collapse of all fished species within fifty years. The ocean will basically be void of fish if we don't change our eating habits.[86]

Roughly twenty percent of all currently threatened and endangered species in the United States are harmed by livestock grazing, and pesticide used both for crops designed for livestock and for human consumption has a devastating effect on wildlife. Scientists at Cornell University estimate that pesticide use is responsible for killing approximately sixty-seven million birds annually.[87] And scientists are now confirming that the disappearance of the honeybee, which could have truly disastrous effects for our entire crop system, is the result of pesticide and fungicide use.[88]

The state of the environment today can certainly trigger that instinct we have to bury our heads in the sand and willfully put on our blinders when we're overwhelmed. Saving the planet can be overwhelming. But rather than concluding that the problem is too big to fix and carrying on as if it didn't exist, while in the meantime contributing to what is a very real crisis, we can approach the issue of the environment like everything else. We start where we are. We educate ourselves enough to make choices that do no harm.

No one is going to save the planet single-handedly. We *can* save the planet as a collective of individuals, taking responsibility for our own actions. Just as world peace must begin with inner peace, a healthy environment must begin with individual stewardship. Ultimately, we can only be responsible for ourselves. That is something we can do, and it is where all change begins. Animal agriculture is the leading threat to the environment today. It follows that giving up animal products in our diet is unquestionably the single most important action we can take to help save our planet. ❀

2

Right Diet as a Way of Life

Beyond the Cleanse

We now have a deep and broad range of evidence showing that a whole foods, plant-based diet provides the best protection against heart disease, cancer, diabetes, and autoimmune diseases (e.g., multiple sclerosis). . . . Furthermore, it turns out that if we eat the way that promotes the best health for ourselves, we promote the best health for the planet. By eating a whole foods, plant-based diet, we use less water, less land, fewer resources and produce less pollution and less suffering for our farm animals. . . . Good nutrition creates health in all areas of our existence. All parts are interconnected.—T. Colin Campbell, Ph.D.[1]

"Right diet" has been understood from the earliest civilizations to be the most important factor in good health. It's the most significant component of Ayurveda, the ancient Indian healing system (discussed below), and an essential element of the Buddha's noble Eightfold Path. What's more, modern nutritional science is now catching up with that ancient wisdom. Right diet reflects the fundamental truth and deep wisdom that Dr. Campbell points to. Our physical health is not separate from our spiritual health; our personal health is not separate from the health of all other living beings and the planet. Our interest in personal health is not at odds with our interest in serving and protecting others and living a life based on ahimsa. Living right and eating right have everything to do with our awakening to the truth of interconnection. What is good for one is good for all.

Diseases of Affluence and *The China Study*

> A low-fat plant-based diet would not only lower the heart attack rate about 85 percent, but would lower the cancer rate 60 percent.—**William Castelli, M.D.**, Director, Framingham Health Study; National Heart, Lung, and Blood Institute[2]

> Five to ten percent of all cancers are caused by inherited genetic mutations. By contrast, 70 to 80 percent have been linked to [diet and other] behavioral factors.—**Karen Emmons, M.D.**, Dana-Farber Cancer Institute, Boston[3]

The illnesses that most affect Americans are the so-called diseases of affluence: heart disease, cancer, type 2 diabetes, obesity, high blood pressure, stroke, autoimmune conditions, and others. These diseases are related to the overconsumption of certain nutrients. Specifically, research shows a high correlation between consuming animal protein and rates of these ailments. But there is reason for hope, as an increasing body of nutritional science shows that a high percentage of these illnesses can be prevented or even reversed by consuming a plant-based diet.

We can acquire all of the nutrients we need from plants without the toxic compounds found in animal-based products. According to Dr. T. Colin Campbell, author of the widely acclaimed *The China Study* (which the *New York Times* called the "Grand Prix of epidemiology" and the "most comprehensive large study ever undertaken of the relationship between diet and the risk of developing disease"), besides the antibiotics, steroids, and hormones that we ingest when we consume the bulk of animal products on the market, "the real danger of animal products is the nutrient imbalances, regardless of the presence or absence of those nasty chemicals. Long before modern chemicals were introduced into our food, people still began to experience more cancer and more heart disease when they started to eat more animal-based foods."[4] In fact, the more animal protein we ingest, the higher the risks of developing these diseases of affluence. *The China Study* makes a compelling health case for giving up animal products.

Dr. Campbell was raised on a dairy farm and grew up believing, as most of us do, that consuming meat and dairy was essential to a healthy life. In 1956, he obtained a bachelor's degree in pre-veterinary medicine from Penn State, and in 1962 he earned a Ph.D. in nutrition, biochemistry, and bacteriology from Cornell University. As he began his career, there was widespread belief that protein was the most important nutrient requirement for human health, and that the lack of it was the most serious nutritional deficiency in the developing world.[5]

He joined a team of researchers involved in international nutrition policy who traveled to the Philippines to launch a program for malnourished children. As he studied the population for protein consumption, he was simultaneously looking at rates of liver cancer, which happened to be very high in the country. It was believed this was caused by consuming aflatoxin, a carcinogen found on peanuts. However, when Dr. Campbell examined the combined data on protein and aflatoxin consumption and cancer he discovered that it wasn't the rate of aflatoxin consumption that drove up cancer rates, it was protein. The research showed that the children of the wealthiest Filipino families who consumed the diets with the most protein were the ones most likely to get liver cancer. The poorer rural children had a lower incidence.

Shortly after his discoveries in the Philippines, Dr. Campbell reviewed a study by Indian researchers that seemed to confirm his unexpected observations in the Philippines. The Indian study compared two groups of rats. The first group was fed twenty percent animal protein, which is about what the average American who's not on a high-protein diet consumes. The second group of rats was fed a diet of five percent animal protein. Both groups were then given an equal amount of aflatoxin.

Every rat in the group who ate the twenty percent animal protein developed cancerous tumors. Not one rat in the five-percent group did.

Not long afterward, Dr. Junshi Chen, a distinguished scientist from China, came to work in Dr. Campbell's lab. Dr. Chen had been in charge of the "Cancer Atlas," a massive survey of 880 million Chinese citizens (ninety-six percent of the population at the time) in 2,400 Chinese counties. The atlas graphically depicted where certain types of cancer were high and where they were almost nonexistent. The map made it clear that cancer rates were geographically determined, to the extreme, with some areas showing more than a hundred times the amount of cancer than other areas. By comparison, in the United States, cancer rates in certain areas might be two or three times higher than other areas, at most. With the atlas as the foundation of their work, Dr. Campbell assembled an international team of scientists and began what would be the first joint research study between the United States and China.

More than 8,000 statistically significant associations were found between various factors and disease. Data were gathered on 365 variables in sixty-five counties across China. Questionnaires were given to 6,500 people along with blood and urine tests. When he analyzed the data, Dr. Campbell found that all the associations pointed to the same findings: the people who ate the most animal protein had the highest rates of cancer and other "lifestyle disease" or "diseases of affluence."

Dr. Campbell went back to the lab and tried to repeat the Indian study. His results were even more compelling because he ran the tests in various stages with different variables. To begin with, he repeated the original study design, separating two groups of mice, feeding them both equal amounts of aflatoxin and then giving one group five percent animal protein (he used casein, which is a protein found in milk), and the other group twenty percent casein. None of the five-percent mice developed tumors; all of the twenty-percent mice did.

In another round, he took the twenty percent group, all of whom had tumors, and switched them to a five percent casein diet. In all cases, the tumors shrank. When he took them back to twenty percent casein, the tumors grew back. The animal protein was like a switch, and he was able to turn the cancer growth on and off through administering animal protein. In later phases, he also experimented with using five versus twenty percent plant protein to determine whether the trigger was simply high protein itself or specifically animal protein. No tumors grew in mice fed a diet of twenty percent plant protein, confirming for Dr. Campbell that the cancer promoter, or trigger, was not just protein but specifically animal protein.

Living Well into Old Age

The Japanese island of Okinawa lies about a thousand miles south of Tokyo. Its residents have one of the world's longest life expectancies, and there are more centenarians there than in any other state or country worldwide. Daily, Okinawans eat an average of seven servings of vegetables, eleven servings of whole grains, and two servings of soy (the highest soy consumption in the world; note, this is unprocessed and non-GMO soy). They eat fish two to three times a week and almost no meat or dairy.

In his book *Healthy at 100*, John Robbins surveyed those populations of people around the globe with the highest percentage of living centenarians. He concluded that their longevity could be attributed to certain commonalities in lifestyle rather than to genetics.[6] Migration research confirms this. For example, in Dr. Campbell's China study, the rates of cancer varied by a hundred times depending on region, even within the same ethnic group, the Han, who comprise the majority of Chinese.

In his research, John Robbins found that the populations scattered across the globe that live the longest are those who eat a mostly plant-based, whole foods diet; are physically active; and have community, and rich, satisfying lives. It's not genetics, and it's not a wonder drug. It's a good life. This good life is not quite the modern Western concept of a good life filled with money, physical beauty, material possessions, and power, but rather one that is rich in family and friendship and involves living in harmony with the natural world.

Plant-Based Nutrition 101

For those of us who grew up in North America, it may be hard to comprehend that not only can we be healthy eating a purely plant-based diet, but we can be among the healthiest people on the planet. The most common question every vegan gets is, "But where do you get your protein?" betraying the common misperception that we need meat, eggs, or dairy in order to get protein, or that somehow we risk starvation without enough of it. When I was first trying to become a vegan, those questions really troubled me. *Where* was *I getting my protein? Was I getting enough? Was I going to wither away from malnutrition?* It's helpful to understand just a few basics about nutrition to put our own doubts to rest.

Protein

Protein is a combination of amino acids. There are twenty standard amino acids, and we need all of them to perform a range of important functions in our bodies, from metabolizing to replicating DNA to muscle development. Plants have the ability to produce all of these on their own, but animals like us can only manufacture eleven by ourselves. We need to obtain the other nine through food. Those we must obtain through food are called "essential" amino acids.

Essential amino acids can be obtained from animals or plants. Most animal flesh is similar to our own and contains all nine essential amino acids in the proportions we need. Most plants also contain all of the essential amino acids, but often are low in one or more of them. So rather than relying on one food source for all of our protein needs, we need to obtain our protein from a range of foods. (This is the origin of the protein-combining myth popularized in the 1970s and that stubbornly persists despite all the scientific evidence to the contrary. According to this myth, because plant-based proteins don't contain all of the right amounts of essential amino acids, we need to combine specific proteins to form perfect, complete proteins with every meal. This would really be a big hassle. Fortunately, it's not true.)

Our bodies are smarter than we realize. They form protein chains out of a pool of amino acids that we collect and store every time we eat. When we need them, the body draws them from that pool. We don't need to combine proteins with every meal. We shouldn't try to live on bananas, lentils, or any single food source; but this principle holds for all humans, not just vegans. No one would want to eat only steak, no matter how perfect its protein, because if that were all we ate, we'd develop a range of other nutritional problems, such as Vitamin C deficiency and a host of conditions related to the lack of fiber in the diet.

It's also the case that many traditional pairings of foods provide the complete set of essential amino acids we need, so more often than not we unintentionally combine proteins anyway. Some examples of these perfect food marriages are a peanut butter sandwich (nuts and grains), or black or red beans and rice. Moreover, both soybeans and quinoa are their own complete proteins, the same as a steak.

The other prevalent myth around protein is that more is better. The average American consumes seventy to a hundred grams of protein a day. The Recommended Dietary Allowance (RDA) as set by the U.S. government is fifty to sixty grams, which is an inflated number because it has to account for populations with higher protein needs, such as pregnant women. But high protein intake is linked to an increase in almost all the diseases of affluence, as well as an increase in the rate of osteoporosis and kidney disease.

The RDA for protein equates to roughly ten to fifteen percent of total calories consumed. But the World Health Organization recommends that only about four to five percent of calories come from protein.[7] Vegans can get plenty of protein in their diet by consuming a variety of beans, seeds, nuts, whole grains, and vegetables, all of which contain protein, and some of which contain a lot of protein. Just one cup of tofu contains about twenty grams of protein, and spinach is fifty-one percent protein. If we're worried we won't get enough protein, we can look to nature for perspective. The largest and strongest land animals on Earth are plant eaters, including the elephant, gorilla, buffalo, hippo, and cow.

Fiber and Complex Carbohydrates

Fiber is essential to good health. It binds to toxins in the body and helps eliminate them. It keeps digestion moving. Without it, we're susceptible to diseases such
as colorectal cancer and large bowel cancer, which are based partly on irregular
or inadequate bowel movements. High fiber consumption reduces the risk of these
and other cancers, lowers blood cholesterol, and is associated with healthy weight.
Dietary fiber is *only* found in plants, not in animal-based foods.

We obtain fiber from fruits, vegetables, and whole grains. For the last couple of
decades, carbohydrates have gotten a bad rap. But not all carbs are created equally.
Whole grains contain not just high fiber but a range of other nutrients such as
protein, vitamins, minerals, and other beneficial compounds found in plants, called
phytonutrients. Whole grains are those intact grains containing the bran, endo-
sperm, and germ.

Refined grains have been stripped of the bran and the germ, and, in the process,
of most of their vitamins and other healthful compounds. We see refined grains as
white flour, processed breads and sweets, pastas, crackers, and most cereals. These
are the "empty calories" that lead to weight gain and exacerbate diseases like diabetes. It's important to distinguish between whole grains and refined grains.

Calcium

As we all know, calcium is important for building healthy bones. However, contrary
to those milk ads (the key word here is "ads") that most of us grew up believing were
some kind of public service announcement, milk is not the only source of calcium;
in fact, it's not even the best source. Cup for cup, leafy greens like collard greens
provide more calcium than milk. Furthermore, many studies show that consuming
milk increases the risk of other diseases, such as cancer and heart disease, as well as
overall mortality. Consuming three glasses of milk a day nearly doubles our mortality rate.[8] Vegans can obtain all the calcium we need by eating leafy greens, such as
collards, kale, and broccoli; legumes like black beans and chickpeas; fortified soy
milk and calcium-set tofu, or taking a 250–300 mg supplement.[9]

Iron

Contrary to popular belief, vegetarians do not have a higher incidence of iron deficiency compared to meat eaters. Remember Popeye? He got his iron, and his strength, from spinach not steak. Vegetarian men, boys, and postmenopausal women shouldn't have to worry about obtaining iron. However, just as in the greater population, premenopausal vegetarian women and teenage girls are more prone to iron deficiency and sometimes even anemia. In order to ensure adequate iron consumption and absorption, follow these simple guidelines:

- Eat lots of dark green leafy vegetables.
- Include a source of vitamin C with meals (which increases absorption of iron).
- Avoid drinking black or green tea (herbal is fine) and coffee with meals (which decreases absorption of iron).
- Incorporate plenty of legumes (peanuts, beans, lentils, peas) into your diet.
- Cook foods in cast-iron skillets.[10]

Antioxidants

Antioxidants prevent oxidation and damage of free radicals at the cellular level. They protect us from cancer, boost immunity, and prevent the destruction of cells. Plants are full of them. All the pigments we see in plants are visual cues that they contain antioxidants. Animals do not produce antioxidants, so we must eat plants to get them.

Vitamin B$_{12}$

The requirement for vitamin B$_{12}$ is very low, but there are no available plant sources of B$_{12}$. B$_{12}$ is found in the soil, and were we to eat our vegetables unwashed we'd get plenty. Most people obtain their B$_{12}$ from animals who get theirs from foraging on grasses. Estimates vary widely, but it's thought that between forty and eighty percent of the general population may be B_{12} deficient, so B_{12} isn't just a concern for vegans. But B_{12} *is* important for proper functioning of the brain and nervous system, so vegans want to include a B_{12} supplement or obtain B_{12} from supplemented foods such as nutritional yeast, fortified soy milk, or meat analogues. Tempeh, miso, and seaweed are often labeled as having large amounts of vitamin B_{12}. However, the amount available varies depending on the type of processing the food has undergone. So it's best to supplement either by taking at least ten micrograms daily, or by taking a weekly B_{12} supplement that provides at least 2,000 micrograms.[11]

The Colors of Health

Phytochemicals, substances found only in plants, act as antioxidants and help our bodies fight disease and promote good health. Phytochemicals can be seen in the pigments of our produce. Each color represents different phytochemicals.

Practically every day we hear a story about a different vitamin we should be taking in order to prevent something terrible from happening. Or there's a new superfood replete with some amazing benefit. In order to actually ingest all of the goji berries, chia seeds, selenium, lycopene (and the list goes on), it sometimes feels like we'd need to stay home and eat all day. Many people turn to supplements and vitamins to try to cram everything good into their bodies in one swallow—like Jane Jetson on her moped in the sky, popping dinner pills. But more and more research indicates that supplements are not only *not* beneficial, they may even be harmful.[12]

The best way to get the full range of vitamins, minerals, and other protective compounds we need is by eating whole foods. And the best way to get the full spectrum and range of those nutrients is to eat a wide variety of whole plant foods. Because the natural pigments in food represent such a variety of nutrients, experts advise eating a wide range of whole foods that span the color spectrum.[13] Here are a few of the health benefits we gain from eating this nutritional rainbow:

Red = Lycopene
Lycopene helps reduce the risk of several types of cancer, including that of the prostate, and may lower the risk of heart and lung diseases. Foods containing these phytochemicals include tomatoes, pink grapefruit, and watermelon.

Yellow/Green = Lutein and Zeaxanthin
Lutein and zeaxanthin are believed to lower the risk of cataracts and age-related macular degeneration. Lutein is a yellow-green substance that concentrates in the back of your eye. It may also reduce the risk of atherosclerosis. Foods in this group include spinach, collard greens, mustard greens, turnip greens, yellow corn, green peas, avocado, and honeydew melon.

Orange = Alpha-Carotene and Beta-Carotene
Alpha-carotene protects against cancer. Beta-carotene, which the body converts to vitamin A, protects the skin against free radical damage and helps repair damaged DNA. Beta-carotene is also good for night vision. Foods in this group include carrots, mangos, apricots, cantaloupe, pumpkin, acorn squash, winter squash, and sweet potatoes.

Orange/Yellow = Beta cryptothanxin, Vitamin C
Beta cryptothanxin helps cells in the body communicate with each other and may help prevent heart disease. Vitamin C protects against immune system deficiencies, cardiovascular disease, prenatal health problems, eye disease, and wrinkles. Foods in this group include pineapple, orange juice, oranges, tangerines, peaches, papayas, and nectarines.

Red/Purple = Anthocyanins

Anthocyanins are powerful antioxidants that help control high blood pressure and protect against diabetes-related circulatory disorders. They are known to have anti-inflammatory properties and are believed to protect against heart disease by preventing blood clots. They may also slow the aging of cells and have been linked to delayed onset of Alzheimer's disease. Foods in this group include beets, eggplant, purple grapes, red wine, grape juice, prunes, cranberries, blueberries, blackberries, strawberries, and red apples.

Green = Sulforaphane, Isocyanate, and Indole

Sulforaphane, isocyanate, and indole all prevent cancer by inhibiting carcinogens. Foods in this group include broccoli, Brussels sprouts, cabbage, Chinese cabbage or bok choi, and kale.

White/Green = Allicin

The onion family contains allicin, an important compound for fighting tumors. Foods in this group include leeks, scallions, garlic, onions, celery, pears, white wine, endive, and chives.

GMOs, Pesticides, and Organics

Genetically modified organisms (GMOs) are plants or animals that are genetically modified with DNA from bacteria, viruses, or other plants and animals. At present, the GMO crops available in the United States are limited to alfalfa (first planting in 2011), canola (approx. ninety percent of U.S. crop), corn (approx. eighty-eight percent of U.S. crop in 2011), cotton (approx. ninety percent of U.S. crop in 2011), papaya (most of the Hawaiian crop; approximately 988 acres), soy (approx. ninety-four percent of U.S. crop in 2011), sugar beets (approx. ninety-five percent of U.S. crop in 2010), zucchini and yellow summer squash (approx. 25,000 acres) and all nonorganic meat and dairy because of feed contamination.[14]

The arguable benefit of such a product is that it's engineered to withstand exposure to various herbicides and pesticides. The basic idea is that we can spray a GMO crop and kill any weeds or pests that might otherwise damage it without harming the crop itself. Theoretically, you could also engineer crops to withstand droughts or contain higher quantities of nutrients, which is why these products were lauded as a "Green Revolution" solution to world hunger.

This noble goal has not translated into reality. A 2009 report overseen by the United Nations, containing the work of more than four hundred scientists and approved by more than fifty countries, questioned the validity of using GMO crops to address food insecurity. Instead, it stressed the existence of more effective alternatives and solutions.[15] As noted above, one such alternative urged by the United Nations, among other international entities, is a global shift toward a plant-based diet in order to save the world from hunger, resource loss, and the worst impacts of climate change.[16]

Whether GMOs could be used in a way that would benefit humanity and alleviate world hunger has little if anything to do with consumption of GMOs in industrialized countries. We certainly have hunger issues in our own backyard, with fifty million Americans reportedly living in food-insecure households in 2011, 33.5 million of them adults and 16.7 million children.[17] But hunger in America has a lot to do with poverty and little if anything to do with crop shortages. Indeed, in the United States thirty to forty percent of food is wasted, which in effect means that each person throws away twenty pounds of edible food each month.[18]

Two decades of under-regulated use of GMOs on our food supply has shown that heavy use of the herbicide glyphosate on Roundup Ready crops (those that can withstand the herbicide Roundup, which is also commonly used on home lawns, gardens, and golf courses) has led to the development of glyphosate-resistant "super-weeds." To deal with them, we're now using even higher amounts of more dangerous herbicides. A report by Charles Benbrook, a research professor at the Center for Sustaining Agriculture and Natural Resources at Washington State University, found that GMO crops have led to an increase in overall pesticide use by 404 million pounds from the time they were first introduced in 1996.[19]

According to researchers at the Massachusetts Institute of Technology (MIT), heavy use of Roundup could be linked to a range of health problems and diseases, including Parkinson's, infertility, and cancers.[20] Many scientists are also concerned that GMOs, once consumed, may pass on their mutated DNA to bacteria in the digestive system.[21] A study released in June 2013 showed that pigs fed GMO crops had significantly increased stomach inflammation.[22]

The moral of the story is, avoid GMOs. This is difficult to do because there is currently no requirement in the United States that GMOs be labeled. Until we pass legislation enforcing labeling, we can avoid GMOs by ensuring that we only purchase organic soy, corn, sugar beets, cotton, alfalfa, squash, and canola oil. What's really sneaky is that sixty to seventy percent of processed foods on U.S. grocery shelves have genetically modified ingredients. But they come in a variety of forms like corn syrup and soy protein isolate, so we have to read our labels carefully.

Pesticides

Of the approximately 84,000 chemicals on the market today, about one percent of them have been studied for safety. Most of us have little awareness of the chemicals we routinely ingest through our food. Many of us take for granted that the government will protect us from toxic chemicals. So it's a little shocking to discover that ninety-three percent of Americans tested by the Centers for Disease Control and Prevention (CDC) had metabolites of chlorpyrifos, a neurotoxic insecticide, in their urine. This chemical is banned from home use because of the health risks it poses to children. It has been linked to neurological, developmental, and autoimmune disorders. Yet it's still used on our food supply. In fact, according to the EPA, in commercial agriculture it remains "one of the most widely used organophosphate insecticides."[23] And this is just one pesticide. The nonprofit Pesticide Action Network North America has a database of all the pesticides commonly used on our food. That database includes hundreds of pesticides. Every time we eat a nonorganic crop, we are ingesting some amount of pesticide, many of which are known carcinogens.

The use of pesticides has allowed farmers to produce much higher yields of many crops. But while the government regulates the amount of residue permitted from any one pesticide, it doesn't limit the number of pesticides used. What makes pesticides toxic or dangerous is a combination of how much we ingest and in what combination, and not just in one serving but cumulatively over our lives. Pesticides become stored in fat cells, so while we may only ingest small amounts of pesticides at one time, their residue can build up in our bodies.

While the European Union takes a precautionary approach to both GMO and regular crops, the regulatory standard in the United States is to approve first, and only if and when there is demonstrated harm will the chemical or product be banned. Oftentimes, however, we don't see the harm until much damage has already been done, and it can take generations for some of the residues from pesticides to disappear from the environment.

For example, the insecticide DDT (dichlorodiphenyltrichloroethane) was one of the main families of insecticides to be used after World War II. Originally developed for chemical warfare, it was found to be a powerful insecticide and was widely used in combating malaria, typhus, and other insect-borne human diseases among both military and civilian populations as well as for insect control in crop and livestock production, and in homes and gardens. The EPA banned it in 1972 because of its adverse environmental effects on wildlife as well as its potential human health risks. DDT was the leading cause of the near extinction of the bald eagle in North America in the 1950s and 1960s as well as the brown pelican and the peregrine falcon. Today, DDT is classified as a probable human carcinogen.

Even though DDT hasn't been used in the United States since 1972, the CDC states that we continue to be exposed to it primarily through our food, specifically dairy milk, as well as domestic and imported produce. Nearly all U.S. residents continue to test positive for DDT's primary breakdown product, dichlorodiphenyl-dichloroethylene (DDE).[24]

Organics

Given the dangers of pesticides and GMOs, eating organic whenever possible is the best choice. But it isn't just a matter of personal health. Organic farming can protect the environment and wildlife, not to mention the one to two million migrant farm workers who harvest these crops. If we worry about our own exposure to pesticides from the relatively small quantities of produce we personally handle and consume, we have to multiply the risks to farm workers exponentially, as they are in constant contact with these dangerous chemicals. The EPA has estimated that every year between ten and twenty thousand farm workers suffer acute pesticide poisoning on the job, and long-term exposure to pesticides can lead to brain and lung damage; cancers of the breast, colon, lung, pancreas, and kidney; birth defects, sterility, and other ailments.[25] We need to remember these workers when we are at the grocery store.

The reality, however, is that organics are expensive. Government subsidies largely go to the monoculture crops of soy and corn and to meat and dairy factories, driving down the cost of the unhealthiest foods, while the cost of fresh, organic produce remains high. So it's helpful to know which foods are most important to buy organic. Besides GMO crops, some crops are "dirtier" than others. The not-for-profit think tank the Environmental Working Group (EWG) issues an annual list, the "Dirty Dozen," which names the crops most contaminated by pesticides in our food supply. These produce items contain the most toxic chemicals most difficult to remove (even when washed diligently).

The list is updated annually. For 2015, the dirty dozen are:

1. Apples
2. Peaches
3. Nectarines
4. Strawberries
5. Grapes
6. Celery
7. Spinach
8. Sweet bell peppers
9. Cucumbers
10. Cherry tomatoes
11. Snap peas—Imported
12. Potatoes[26]

The EWG also compiles a list of the cleanest fruits and vegetables, the "Clean Fifteen." These are items that have the lowest pesticide residue and are therefore the safest to buy conventionally farmed (i.e., nonorganic). These are:

1. Avocados
2. Sweet Corn
3. Pineapples
4. Cabbage
5. Sweet peas (frozen)
6. Onions
7. Asparagus
8. Mangos
9. Papayas
10. Kiwi
11. Eggplant
12. Grapefruit
13. Cantaloupe
14. Cauliflower
15. Sweet Potatoes[27]

We all have cells in our bodies that could grow into tumors, but we don't all develop cancer. The reason is that there needs to be something that triggers those cells to form tumors. As discussed, Dr. Campbell's research indicates that animal protein is a pervasive and powerful trigger. So eating a plant-based diet will go a long way to protecting us from the inevitable exposure. In addition, eating foods that boost our immune systems, foods that are high in antioxidants and linked to cancer prevention (plants!), can help us prevent the growth of unhealthy cells.

However, even if we live at the top of a secluded, pristine mountain, we cannot escape exposure to a barrage of carcinogens and other chemicals in our modern world. If we try to control the things we cannot change, we'll make ourselves crazy as well as sick. Balance lies in our ability to make mindful choices. If we find we're becoming hooked by fear of what we eat, we may need to let go a little bit. Fear is a potent toxin in itself. Health is determined by many different factors; diet is key, but it isn't the only factor to consider. Our state of mind is a powerful component of health. As we integrate all of the information about the food we eat, it's important to stay connected to all of our practices so that our focus will remain on harmony rather than fear.

Ayurveda—The Science of Longevity

Ayurveda is the ancient Indian science of longevity. The forest-dwelling sages or *rishis* of the Himalayas who handed down the traditions of Ayurveda were scientists who practiced deep meditation and observation in order to understand the internal and the external worlds. These sages gave us the seminal Indian spiritual texts such as the *Vedas*. Ayurveda traces its origins to these sacred texts.

The focus of Ayurveda is on the health of the physical body, disease prevention and healing, and maximizing one's lifespan and quality of life. However, its wisdom is deeply connected with an understanding of the interconnectedness of life as a whole. Ayurveda views the human being as a complex, interrelated combination of physical/mental/spiritual traits, which cannot be separated. Not only are all of these parts of ourselves connected, but as Indian-originated philosophies such as yoga and Buddhism teach us, we're connected to all other living beings and the environment. When any one of these parts is out of harmony with the other, we experience suffering.

According to Ayurveda, right lifestyle is the foundation of a healthy, harmonious life in mind, body, and spirit, which honors the interconnection of all life.[28] An essential part of right lifestyle is right diet, which is considered the main component of healing the physical body.[29] Ayurveda tells us that when we treat the body as separate from the mind and the spirit, disease arises. Seeing ourselves as discrete individuals with no connection to the world on the other side of our skin is a primary mark of *maya*, the veil of ignorance and illusion. Maya refers to the fundamentally limited and distorted way we perceive the world, preventing us from seeing ultimate truth.

In Plato's *Republic*, the Greek philosopher presents his "Allegory of the Cave," which illustrates the nature of our illusion. In his allegory, Plato describes prisoners who live chained to the wall of a cave with their backs to the entrance. On the wall in front of them shadows appear, formed by the figures passing in front of a fire behind them. The cave dwellers watch the shadows and take them for reality. One day, one of the prisoners is freed. He leaves the cave and walks into the sunlight.

Blinded at first, his eyes soon acclimate to the light and he sees the world as it truly is. With his newfound insight, he returns to the cave to tell the others that the shadows aren't real, but the cave dwellers, knowing no other reality, think the free man has gone insane. Like the cave dwellers, we live under an illusion of separation, believing we're separated from one another by the boundaries of our physical bodies.

Like Eastern philosophy, modern science confirms that much of our basic understanding of reality is simply wrong. For example, when we look at our own bodies we see a solid distinct mass. I sit in a chair and I assume I am making contact with that chair. Why wouldn't I? Yet science tells us that in fact neither I, nor my chair, is solid. Rather, we are a collection of constantly moving atoms, each composed of over 99.99 percent space, exactly like the universe. As I type this, and you read this, neither of us is really sitting on our chairs but rather hovering over them, the electrons surrounding our atoms repelling each other to create the illusion that we are making contact.

But, of course, though neither I nor the wall in front of me are solid in the way I perceive us to be, if I were to run headfirst into that wall, the pain I'd feel would appear awfully real. Understanding ultimate reality doesn't exempt us from the laws of relative reality.

Similarly, Eastern philosophy holds that our fundamental ignorance (*avidya*) of the nature of ultimate reality both within and without is the root cause of all of our suffering, whether psychological or physical. Although deeply rooted in an understanding of this ultimate reality, or ultimate wisdom, Ayurveda deals directly with the relative reality in which we find ourselves, and with our bodies and world as we actually experience both.

Accordingly, a hallmark of the Ayurvedic system is its recognition that all individuals are just that: individual. What works for one person may wreak havoc on another person's constitution. While working within some general parameters such as those discussed below, we're advised to pay attention to our own bodies and heed the prodding of our own intuition. For example, if spicy foods don't agree with us, we should avoid them; if raw foods make us sick, we should cook our food.

It's important that we enjoy what we eat and properly digest our food in order to feel healthy and vibrant. If we have trouble digesting certain plant-based foods, it can sabotage our attempts to adopt a plant-based diet and impede our ability to enjoy all the potential benefits of the diet. If we're not digesting properly we won't absorb all the nutrients available, either. So we must choose the right foods and prepare them in the right way for ourselves as individuals with different constitutions. Ayurveda helps us find what works best for us as individuals.

The basic Ayurvedic view is that all individuals are comprised of a mixture of three basic *doshas* or forces: *Vata*, *Pitta*, and *Kapha*, which correspond to the combined elements of air and ether, fire and water, and earth and water respectively. When any one of the doshas is out of balance, illness or disease occurs. All individuals have a basic type—pure Vata, pure Pitta, pure Kapha, or some combination. Ayurveda is the science of balancing the doshas. This is accomplished through a range of practices, but right diet is the primary tool for bringing the body into alignment.

While Ayurveda, as I've argued, is a highly individualized science, some general principles apply to all the doshas:

- No one can properly digest food when stressed out. We should always eat when calm and in a comfortable environment.
- We should eat with people who make us feel comfortable.
- We shouldn't eat food prepared by anyone who doesn't love us. This means that we ought to minimize how much we eat out.
- We shouldn't overeat. Eat only the amount you can hold in your cupped hands.
- When we eat, half the stomach should be filled with solid food, a quarter with liquids, and a quarter left empty.
- We should only eat after completely digesting the previous meal.

Another of Ayurveda's central teachings is that we all have an inner healer. We only need to tap into this wisdom and become aware of what our bodies and our hearts tell us. People of different doshas react differently to the same foods. So, for example, a Pitta has the capacity to digest kidney beans without intestinal distress, whereas a Vata will likely suffer terrible indigestion from the same bean. We probably already know on some level which foods agree with us and which don't, whether we feel better eating a very raw diet or more cooked food. We probably have some sense of how many hours a night we need to sleep in order to feel rested and stay healthy. But maybe we ignore what we sense for a number of reasons. Our yoga teacher tells us that a raw diet is the healthiest way to eat, so we force ourselves to eat raw because we think she probably knows more than we do, despite the fact that we aren't digesting any of that raw food so it can't actually do us any good. Or we can't get the amount of sleep we feel we need because our partner sleeps less and wakes us up, so we just try to deal with it.

More than anything, Ayurveda tells us to pay attention and trust our own bodies; this is what makes it so compelling. It reinforces our own instincts, our own wisdom. It teaches us that our innate wisdom is important and we shouldn't discount it. How many times do we say to ourselves, *I should stop now; I'm totally not hungry anymore* and then we get an extra piece of pizza or slice of cake? And then we feel bad, but we continue to do it anyway because we get stuck in that cycle of looking for happiness outside of ourselves. It seems we are endlessly trying to fill that spiritual craving with non-spiritual substances that can never reach the true source of our thirst. The longer we stay stuck in these habits/patterns, the more likely we are to develop illness or disease.

Most of us are also likely to experience confusion over all the conflicting health information we come across. Ayurveda tells us we have the answers we need within. It provides us with a lot of ancient wisdom but ultimately leaves it to us to determine what works and what doesn't. In fact, this is how we self-determine what our dosha is and accordingly what we need to do to achieve optimal health.

In order to determine your specific dosha, you can consult with an Ayurvedic doctor or find one of the many dosha tests available online or in almost any book you might purchase on Ayurveda. A couple of general indicators of your dosha are your temperature and climate preferences, as well as your general emotional impulses. For example, if you're very sensitive to heat, you're probably Pitta. If it's not heat but humidity that oppresses you, you're likely Kapha. If you love heat of any kind, you're probably Vata. When we're trying to identify our doshas, it's most helpful to look at our lifelong tendencies, more than where we are right now.

Our emotional tendencies can reveal our doshas as well. If you were sitting at your kitchen table early in the morning reading the newspaper and drinking tea and you heard a noise at your front door, how would you (most likely) instinctively react? A Vata would scream with fear or maybe call 911, if she weren't too anxious about whether or not calling was the right thing to do (because Vatas also vacillate quite a lot and are prone to self-doubt). If your first reaction would be anger or annoyance, like, *Who the &#@! is at my door this early in the morning while I'm trying to enjoy some peace and tranquility?!* or you're ready to grab a bat and go at the intruder, you're probably a Pitta. If you tell yourself there's nothing there and try to distract yourself, denying what's happening altogether, you're probably a Kapha.

Vata is associated with motion. Vatas tend to have a lot of nervous energy that keeps them running from one place to another. For this reason, a lot of motion, including too much travel or staying too busy, also imbalances them. Vatas are often cold and dry. They can also be or feel rather flighty or "spacey." They have the weakest digestion of the three doshas and so need more spices, like ginger, in their diet to stimulate the digestive fire.

Pitta is associated with transformation. Pittas have a fiery temperament. They may be prone to anger and can be very passionate. They're generally in good shape physically but overheat easily and prefer cooler climates. With fire as their element, Pittas have the strongest digestive fire, which is why, for example, they can eat those red beans and rice with no trouble.

Kapha is associated with stability. Kaphas are the homebodies. Sensitive and emotional, when imbalanced they may be prone to depression. They don't seek drama, like Pittas do, but are peaceful. While both Vata and Pitta are light in nature, Kapha is heavy. These qualities of heaviness and stability incline Kaphas toward being overweight.

General Guidelines for Balancing Vata Dosha
- Keep warm
- Eat warming foods and spices
- Keep calm
- Establish and maintain a regular routine
- Get plenty of rest
- Avoid cold, frozen, or raw foods
- Avoid extreme cold

General Guidelines for Balancing Pitta Dosha
- Avoid excessive heat
- Eat cooling, non-spicy foods
- Avoid excessive oil
- Exercise during the coolest part of the day
- Avoid excessive humidity
- Limit salt intake

General Guidelines for Balancing Kapha Dosha
- Stay active and get plenty of exercise
- Vary your routine
- Avoid fatty, oily, and heavy foods
- Eat light meals, including raw or lightly cooked ingredients
- Avoid dairy
- Avoid daytime naps
- Avoid iced foods and drinks

How Food Influences the Mind: Sattvic, Rajasic, *and* Tamasic *Foods*
According to the *Samkhya* philosophy in which both Ayurveda and yoga are rooted, the whole manifest physical world, including our own minds, is made up of three basic properties or qualities, called the *gunas*. A predominantly *sattvic* mind is

harmonious, balanced, and tranquil; a *rajasic* mind is busy and characterized by lots of activity and disturbance; an overly *tamasic* mind is dull and lethargic. Foods, too, embody these qualities, with certain foods promoting one or the other.

Ayurveda is used to prevent and treat illness in the body; therefore, certain foods with medicinal qualities that aren't otherwise sattvic may be used. For example, garlic and onions are considered rajasic because they're so stimulating. From an Ayurvedic perspective they can be very healing, just as they are known to be by modern nutritional science.

In general, spiritual seekers are advised to eat a highly sattvic diet to promote harmony within us but also with the entire animal kingdom and the environment. The food is organically grown, vegetarian, sweet, freshly prepared, whole, natural, lightly cooked or seasoned, and not overly spiced or oily. The diet promotes lightness in the body, and is full of *prana* or universal energy. Sattvic foods are easy to digest. They bring clarity and heighten perception, and so are ideal for when we're

Note on Dairy

Ayurveda discourages eating meat and eggs but dairy has traditionally been considered a sattvic food. This tradition, however, dates back to a time and place when cows were revered as sacred and cared for by individuals, not corporations, as a form of religious devotion, under circumstances where calves nursed from their mothers and cows lived out their natural lifespans. As Ayurvedic doctor David Frawley says, the benefit of milk comes from the love of the cow for her calf. But when the calf is separated from his mother, or she is living in miserable and unsanitary conditions (as is the case on most of the dairy farms where milk comes from today), the milk loses its healthful benefits and can no longer be considered sattvic. "All foods produced by harming living beings are to be avoided."[30]

engaging in a lot of meditation. If we notice we're struggling to calm the mind in our yoga or meditation practice, it can be helpful to incorporate more sattvic foods into the diet. A sattvic diet avoids processed, canned, or frozen foods, and should be prepared with love. Some examples of sattvic foods include most fruits such as mango, pomegranate, coconut, figs, peaches, and pears; grains such as rice and blue corn; vegetables such as sweet potato, lettuce, parsley, sprouts, and yellow squash; beans like mung, yellow lentils, kidney, and lima.

Rajasic foods are hot, spicy, and salty. They are stimulating and thus disturb the body and the mind, though they may be tempting and delicious. They are also oily, though not necessarily fatty. It's often more the spicing and the preparation of foods, rather than the foods themselves, that determine their dominant quality; but some examples of rajasic foods include garlic, onions, leeks, coffee and tea, alcohol, artificially sweetened foods, and energy drinks. (If you're concerned with cancer prevention, it would be advisable to retain the allium family of vegetables in your diet—including garlic and onions, which have powerful anticancer properties.)

Tamasic foods are heavy, fatty, fermented, no longer fresh, fried, or difficult to digest. Foods prepared while the cook is angry or filled with negative emotions are also considered tamasic. Tamasic foods include meat, poultry, fish, eggs, alcohol, tobacco, onions, garlic, fermented foods (such as vinegar), and stale, rotten, or over-ripe foods. Tamasic foods are seen to promote disease and ignorance and should be avoided.

Ayurvedic Lifestyle

When we practice any one of the spiritual teachings deeply, we come to see how interconnected all of the teachings are. When we choose right diet, we end up adopting many other practices such as ahimsa and saucha, as we harm many fewer living beings for our food, and we purify our own bodies through the clean foods we eat. While right diet is central to Ayurvedic healing, it's important not to forget that right diet is a part of right lifestyle. Sattvic living, or right lifestyle, includes the purity that comes from eating the right diet, but also that which comes from exercising and from purifying the mind through ahimsa, satya, and compassion for all beings. Right lifestyle also involves practices that connect us to the Divine, such as yoga and meditation, and also right livelihood, an essential tenet of the noble Eightfold Path as taught by the Buddha.

Right livelihood means earning a living in a way that causes no harm to any living being or to the planet. It implies making a living without compromising our values, without violating our ethics, earning a paycheck without lying, without taking what does not belong to us, without greed. Traditionally, it has meant not profiting off of killing, whether by helping to manufacture guns or butchering animals for meat. It also means not price gouging our customers just because we can, and being fair and honest in all of our dealings. In today's world, it also must include a commitment not to harm the Earth. More than doing no harm, right livelihood culminates in our commitment to doing something with our lives that goes beyond non-harming and has a net positive impact in the world, by reducing the suffering of living beings and protecting the planet.

Ayurveda says true health and wellness come when we're living in a state of harmony with the whole of nature. We can become sick both when our physical habits are unhealthy and also when our spiritual lives are deficient in some way. Dr. David Frawley says sickness can arise when we're "not living up to our spiritual purpose or in life, not following our Dharma."[31]

I learned this lesson the hard way.

I always knew I wanted to do something with my life to help the planet. I went to law school with lofty ideas that I'd use my degree for noble intentions. For a host of reasons, however, when I graduated I didn't have that save-the-world job I'd hoped for lined up. I discovered that all the nonprofits I wanted to work for either couldn't afford to pay me or wanted someone with more experience. So I went to work for the government to acquire those skills. Then I got stuck there acquiring the wrong set of skills. Almost every day I felt I was wasting my life. Five years out of law school I was actually more in debt than I was when I'd first graduated.

Under the crushing weight of law-school loans, I took a job with a big law firm working in the food and drug group, where our clients were primarily large pharmaceutical companies. There was no question when I took the job that I had ethical conflicts representing these corporations. In my interview with a partner who knew of my animal rights leanings, I was warned I wouldn't be allowed to take part in any protests against our clients, even if they were testing on animals or engaging in other practices with which I didn't agree. I went home after that interview indignant and determined to turn the job offer down with an unequivocal and righteous diatribe that I wouldn't sell my soul and work for anyone who put profit ahead of morality. Then I went for a haircut a few days later and my credit card was declined because I was over my limit and my bank account was empty. I broke down and, defeated, accepted the job.

I remember visiting one of the clients' offices one day to meet with sales reps to talk about off-label marketing of pharmaceuticals. The manager who met me at the front led me through the building. "Sales is down here . . . and legal is in that wing . . . and that's where we do R&D." R&D, or Research and Development, is where drugs are tested on nonhuman animals. I was sick to my stomach and felt I would cry right there. I was distracted the rest of the day and angry with myself for what felt like having sold my soul. As soon as I was able to leave the building, I cried in the parking lot.

Besides animal testing, I knew my work directly supported an industry that I believed represents much of what is wrong with our modern Western approach to health. This was clear every time I watched a partner eat steak at lunch and follow it with one of the cholesterol pills made by the companies we represented. I knew Big Pharma executives were getting rich off their patented drugs while throughout the world many people were dying from diseases that could have been treated by these same medicines. This wasn't what I wanted to devote my life to; this wasn't my purpose on Earth. I was depressed, sick all the time, and embarrassed to tell people what I did for a living. But I was too scared to let go of the job security and the paycheck.

At first, I worked diligently to please the demanding partners, attempting to prove my worth to them and to myself. In a fairly short span of time, however, I began to resent the work as well as the law-firm culture. I was also becoming consumed by a personal drama in my life. I was engaged to a habitually relapsing drug addict. I had no spiritual practice and no real tools to deal with the chaos that addiction and codependence bring. I stopped seeking out work and sat in my office behind a closed door hoping no one would bring any to me. Therefore, it wasn't a surprise when, in 2008, I was one of a number of associates let go.

I'd been warned several times that I needed to bolster my billable hours or succumb to the layoffs sweeping through the whole legal community. In one of these meetings, the head partner in my group told me I needed to "compartmentalize" my personal issues, and when I began to cry in his office I remember him handing me a bottle of water, which seemed a futile (albeit well-intentioned) gesture. In truth, being laid off was exactly what I needed. I'd been too afraid to take the plunge on my own. As I sat across from the HR person who gave me the official news, I remember struggling to keep a straight face as the ridiculous but joyous image ran through my mind of a frog in a pink tutu leaping euphorically across a stage. I was finally free of the sham.

They say it is the stumble that throws us forward. I've found this to be true. I'm grateful for the stumble and where it threw me. Although it took me some time to land on my feet, since then I've created an entirely different life, one that carries meaning for me and feels aligned with my own purpose. My life is based on serving all living beings and the planet rather than destructive corporate interests and my own self-centered personal and material desires.

I've stopped hiding who I am and how I feel about the world. I live authentically. Little by little, I have brought my livelihood and my life into sync with my values and my heart, which has allowed for the natural expansion and personal evolution that comes when we're true to ourselves. I know firsthand how frightening it can be to let go of a comfortable and seemingly secure life with a large paycheck. And we do need to put all that plant-based food on the table, pay our rent, and cover the vet bills. But to spend our lives clinging to the false security of an unfulfilling career and material wealth is the real impoverishment, one that leads to both personal and global sickness. It takes courage (or sometimes a push) to choose to live simply and in moderation, devoted to a higher purpose and the greater good. It takes heart.

In the words of Carlos Castaneda, this is the important question we need to ask ourselves:

> Does this path have a heart? All paths are the same: they lead nowhere. They are paths going through the bush, or into the bush. In my own life I could say I have traversed long, long paths, but I am not anywhere. . . . Does this path have a heart? If it does, the path is good; if it doesn't, it is of no use. Both paths lead nowhere; but one has a heart, the other doesn't. One makes for a joyful journey; as long as you follow it, you are one with it. The other will make you curse your life. One makes you strong; the other weakens you.[32]

Holistic Weight Loss and Mindfulness

Mindfulness is the best diet in the world. Through mindfulness we can achieve and maintain a healthy weight without force, anxiety, or counting calories. If we are educated and apply what we know, we'll naturally find the right diet that leads to our own healthy weight.

About twenty-three percent of women reported being on a diet in 2012. One in four Americans eats at a fast food restaurant every day. One in every three children born in the year 2000 will develop diabetes in their lifetime. According to the Centers for Disease Control and Prevention, almost seventy percent of Americans are overweight, with about half of them being obese. At the current rate, obesity will soon eclipse smoking as the leading cause of preventable death in the United States. Obesity has been linked to hypertension; coronary heart disease; adult-onset diabetes; stroke; gall bladder disease; osteoarthritis; sleep apnea; respiratory problems; endometrial, breast, prostate, and colon cancers; dyslipidemia; steatohepatitis; insulin resistance; breathlessness and asthma; hyperuricemia; reproductive hormone abnormalities; polycystic ovarian syndrome; impaired fertility; and lower back pain.[33]

On the other end of the spectrum is the widespread obsession with thinness, which leads eleven million Americans to starve themselves, many to death. One in two hundred American women suffers from anorexia; two to three in a hundred American women suffer from bulimia. A study by the National Association of Anorexia Nervosa and Associated Disorders reported that five to ten percent of anorexics die within ten years of contracting the disease; eighteen to twenty percent of anorexics will be dead after twenty years; and only thirty to forty percent ever fully recover. According to the Eating Disorder Coalition, "dieting, a normalized behavior in our culture, is a risk factor for the development of an eating disorder and can trigger eating disorders in those with a genetic predisposition."[34]

Balance comes from shifting our focus away from the appearance of the body to its health. We can also learn from Ayurveda that there is no one-size-fits-all body type. Some people are ideally healthy at a weight that falls far below what the healthy weight range established by the government is, while recent research shows that many people now considered overweight may actually live longer than people considered to have normal body weight.[35]

The true test of the healthiest weight for each of us is what we weigh when we're living healthy, mindful lives: i.e., engaging in daily physical activity; eating a plant-based diet that emphasizes whole foods—including vegetables, fruits, whole grains, seeds, nuts, and beans; and avoiding processed foods, added fats, added sugars, and animal products. If we're living mindful lives, we're much more likely to make the right choices for ourselves. We're more likely to choose whole, unprocessed foods and to stop eating when we're satiated, rather than eating to fill a void that will never be filled with food. We're more likely to stay physically and mentally active and use the tools we have to manage the inevitable stress involved with being alive. Through mindful living, we'll naturally discover our ideal body weight, without the anxiety and struggle that comes from fixating on the result and counting calories or measuring portions.

Of course, in theory it's possible to make really bad choices with full awareness. Theoretically, for example, someone might with full knowledge walk into a grocery store and purposefully head straight for the meat counter and, under the migraine-inducing aura of fluorescent lights, pick up a plastic-wrapped package of greenish-looking chicken breast emblazoned with a label that reads something like:

> WARNING: This product contains body parts of a sentient being who was maimed without anesthesia; confined in an unsanitary, windowless, and overcrowded shed with no access to the outdoors for the duration of his short seven-week life, by which time genetic manipulation had already made it impossible for his own bones to support his unnatural body weight; and then possibly boiled alive because no federal laws protect birds from inhumane slaughter. This product also likely contains arsenic from the feed he was given and is likely contaminated with the deadly e-coli parasite found in feces, as well as steroids, hormones, and antibiotics leading to antibiotic-resistant superbugs. Please cook well.

Although we won't find such a label on the actual package, if we're mindful, that label exists in our minds. Once we become aware of where our food comes from, of the impact it has on the more than nine billion animals killed in America annually for our food, and the impact it has on the planet and on our own lives, we begin to lose our appetite for the standard American diet. No one has to stand over us at the counter and tell us that we'll get fat if we eat the chicken fingers. With mindfulness, we no longer want to eat them.

Most of us would say we don't want to know how our food gets to the plate, because in truth we already *do* know, and it disturbs us. There is practically a species-wide willful blindness about our diet and the impact of our diet for us all. We're so uncomfortable with our diets that we use euphemisms for just about everything we eat, which is a real testament to the power of language. If I call the flesh on my plate "meat" or "hamburger" or "steak," it becomes a senseless object limited in qualities to its taste and texture. However, if I call it what it really is, a body part of a dead cow, I can no longer disassociate the texture and taste from the complex sensitive and emotional living being the bloody mess on my plate once was. We cannot live mindful lives and continue to put our blinders on just for dinner.

Bringing Mindfulness into Our Lives

Mindfulness implies an awareness of reality, an engagement with things as they really are, and a remembrance of our values. When we first begin working with mindfulness, we may only be able to practice it in discrete, structured settings, like during a formal seated meditation practice; or a yoga class or walking meditation practice, where we concentrate on keeping ourselves alert to the present moment. Eventually, we begin to expand our mindfulness practice to the point that it's just how we view the world. And we realize that every single aspect of our lives benefits from the practice. We engage in many pre-eating mindfulness practices. We're mindful about where we shop, possibly selecting the market with the most organic or local produce, and when we get to the grocery store we're mindful about what we put in our carts. The more informed we are, the more aware we can be, and our choices will constantly improve as we continue to learn.

Eating itself can be a very challenging time to practice mindfulness, as we often either eat with companions and talk throughout the meal—totally distracted by the social interaction going on while we shovel food into our mouths—or if alone, we may eat in front of a television or the Internet. Our minds are often scattered as we eat, so we tend to miss out on much of the sensory experience of eating itself.

That said, eating can also be a perfect opportunity for mindfulness. When we do eat mindfully, we transform the experience to such a degree that we begin to choose healthier, more sustainable, and humane foods based on preference rather than repression. We take more enjoyment in our food, as we're more tuned in to the flavors and the colors, and more focused on the pleasure these bring. Our sensations are heightened and the intensity of the enjoyment increases. Because we derive so much enjoyment from each bite, we're satisfied and satiated with much less food and so we're less likely to overeat.

If I'm sitting in front of the TV and petting my dog while simultaneously checking Facebook and eating a chocolate bar, I'm likely to eat half the bar without even realizing I've done it. At that point, I would feel terribly deprived if I had to set it down without even having enjoyed it. How fair would that be? *I've consumed how much fat, sugar, and calories and didn't even notice it!? No way. I'm going back in for more*, and I'll probably only notice that first bite, then again revert to mindlessly feeding myself as I stare blankly at the television until the rest of the bar is gone. At which point, I'll tear open the wrapper in case I've somehow overlooked one last square hiding in the corner because I really can't believe I just ate that whole thing.

Alternatively, I might turn off the television and the computer, give my dog a (vegan) bone and ask him to entertain himself for a while as I sit in silence. With no distractions, I'll focus all of my senses on the square of (fair trade) chocolate I put into my mouth. As I place the chocolate on my tongue, I close my eyes and allow the chocolate to melt just enough that my taste buds dilate and absorb an intensifying flavor that coats and fills my whole mouth. I chew slowly, completely. I am right here, right now, with my chocolate, completely focused, with one-pointed concentration. This is yoga. Mindful eating is not a sacrifice.

Everything we experience is colored by our mindset and our level of attention. When we eat mindfully, we eat the right foods in the right amounts, without force or anxiety. We just do it because it feels right. Therefore, we create no tension, no struggle, and no resistance. When we live healthfully, we are healthy. And "dieting" becomes irrelevant. If we're mindful, we will discover that many of our unhealthy eating habits, along with other unhealthy behaviors, begin to fall away naturally, and in time we achieve the weight that is right for us.

In order to bring mindfulness to the table, it's helpful to pause before we eat and take a second to breathe into the present moment. We might also want to be thankful for the food we eat and to remember those who aren't so fortunate. Eating a plant-based diet allows us to engage reality without anxiety, as the food we eat honors ourselves and all life. Each meal becomes a devotional practice that reconnects us once more with the Divine.

There is a beautiful meal blessing, The Five Contemplations, composed by Thich Nhat Hanh, which can help us eat mindfully and remember the impact of our dietary choices:

- This food is a gift of the earth, the sky, numerous living beings and much hard and loving work.
- May we eat with mindfulness and gratitude so as to be worthy to receive this food.
- May we recognize and transform unwholesome mental formations, especially our greed and learn to eat with moderation.
- May we keep our compassion alive by eating in such a way that reduces the suffering of living beings, stops contributing to climate change, and heals and preserves our precious planet.
- We accept this food so that we may nurture our brotherhood and sisterhood, build our Sangha and nourish our ideal of serving all living beings.[36]

Food Justice

Right diet is about more than just what or what not to eat. It's about being as mindful as possible of the impact all our choices have not just on ourselves but on the world at large. Besides the impact our food choices have on farmed animals, the environment, and our own health, they can shape the structure and power allocations of the society we live in. They link us to numerous beings whose work makes it possible for us to eat, and to numerous other beings in our own communities and around the globe whose lives are impacted by what we choose to eat. The food justice movement encompasses all of these diversely connected issues, including the rights of agricultural workers; depletion of natural resources; the unavailability of healthy foods in communities of color and low-income areas often referred to as "food deserts"; child labor in the global chocolate and coffee industries; and sustainable palm-oil sourcing, among other issues. Although we'll never have perfect knowledge, the more aware we are of the ramifications of our choices, the more we'll be able to live a life that accords with our values and brings us into harmony with other beings.

Farm Workers

We have already touched on pesticides and their effect on farm workers. Unfortunately, this is only one area where farm workers are forgotten. Consider this: "Every time we sit at a table to enjoy the fruits and grain and vegetables from our good earth, remember that they come from the work of men and women and children who have been exploited for generations."[37] Sadly, this statement is as true today as it was when Cesar Chavez, the great labor and civil rights leader, made it years ago. From low wages to dangerous and degrading work conditions, farm laborers are some of the most oppressed members of our society.

Farm workers are specifically excluded from two of the most important federal labor laws. Under the National Labor Relations Act employers are forbidden from firing a worker for joining, organizing, or supporting a labor union. The act also establishes a structure for unions and employers to engage in collective bargaining. Farm workers are excluded from this law. The Fair Labor Standards Act (FLSA), enacted in 1938, guarantees a minimum wage for each hour worked and requires overtime pay for those working more than forty hours in a week. Farm workers have no right to overtime pay; workers on small farms are not entitled to minimum wage; and children as young as twelve are legally allowed to work in the fields.[38]

Female farm workers are arguably the most exploited in the entire workforce. They receive lower pay and are more likely to be laid off. They face all of the same conditions of their male coworkers but confront unique gender issues. A full ninety percent of female farm workers surveyed reported experiencing sexual harassment and discrimination, which often led to rape.[39] We can help improve conditions for farm workers by buying organic, by purchasing Union Label products and products under agreements with farm worker groups such as Farm Labor Organizing Committee (FLOC), Coalition of Immokalee Workers (CIW), and United Farm Workers of America (UFW).[40]

Slaughterhouse Workers

Conditions in slaughterhouses are even worse, where personnel are paid low wages for one of the most physically dangerous workplaces in America. Employees are expected to kill and dismember animals as quickly as possible, which inevitably leads to a range of injuries. As one worker stated, "The line is so fast there is no time to sharpen the knife. The knife gets dull and you have to cut harder. That's when it really starts to hurt, and that's when you cut yourself."[41] Furthermore, the meat packing industry is known for hiring undocumented immigrants who are less likely to assert their legal rights for fear of calling attention to their legal status.[42] Employers take advantage of these fears and use them to routinely violate workers' labor and human rights.[43] And though the research has been slow to emerge, it really should come as no surprise that slaughterhouse workers also suffer a terrible emotional toll from spending their days killing and dismembering other sentient beings. One former slaughterhouse employee put it like this:

> The worst thing, worse than the physical danger, is the emotional toll. . . . Pigs down on the kill floor have come up and nuzzled me like a puppy. Two minutes later I had to kill them—beat them to death with a pipe. I can't care.[44]

Increasingly, slaughterhouse workers are being treated for post-traumatic stress disorder (PTSD), which results from this sort of emotional disassociation. Research confirms that killing sentient beings for a living leads to increased rates of domestic violence, social withdrawal, drug and alcohol abuse, and severe anxiety.[45] In order to perpetuate the industry, we are all forced—to the measure that we are connected to it—to shut off our compassion, our "humanity," and all higher instincts of what is right and decent. The closer we are to it, the more degraded we become. Every time we sit down to a meal, we make a decision about whether we support the grinding debasement of this brutal industry. With every plant-based meal we consume, we help put an end to hell on Earth.

The Chocolate Industry—Not So Sweet

Chocolate is known to contain certain properties that when eaten increase levels of the calming neurotransmitter serotonin as well as the bliss-inducing dopamine. Eating chocolate makes us feel good. But the chocolate industry has a seriously noxious side that our neurotransmitters don't grasp. Western African countries, mostly Ghana and Ivory Coast, supply more than seventy percent of the world's cocoa, used to make chocolate, a $60-billion global industry.[46] Most of us would never imagine that our chocolate was most likely harvested by a child laborer or even a child slave. As far back as 2001, reports of child trafficking and slavery surfaced, prompting some U.S. lawmakers to push for regulations and guarantees to end slavery from the world's largest chocolate producers, but the industry pushed back. The proposed legislation never passed, and the "voluntary agreements" the industry did accept have not been enforced.[47]

As child trafficking and slavery goes on, the industry continues to supply the world's major chocolate producers like Hershey's, Mars, and Nestlé. In 2013, three young men from the African nation of Mali won the right to pursue a case against Archer Daniels Midland (ADM), Cargill, and Nestlé, alleging that they were twelve to fourteen years old when they were first compelled to work as child slaves in cocoa plants belonging to the corporate giants. The plaintiffs said they were forced, often at gunpoint, to work twelve- to fourteen-hour days with no pay. According to their lawyers, they "were given only the bare minimum of food scraps and were locked in small rooms at night with other child slaves so they could not escape the planta-tions. They were whipped and beaten by the guards and overseers when the guards felt they were not working quickly or adequately."[48] In court documents, one of the plaintiffs alleged, "I tried to run away but I was caught . . . as punishment they cut my feet and I had to work for weeks while my wounds healed."[49] Reports of child slavery like these in the cocoa, cotton, and coffee industries are well documented by international nongovernmental organizations (NGOs) like the United Nations[50] and the U.S. State Department.[51]

When we consider the real costs of chocolate, we realize that the "cheap" chocolate tempting us at the checkout aisle isn't cheap at all. The costs are enormous and have been externalized onto powerless children who are robbed of their time, labor, innocence, and freedom. Until the industry is regulated in any real way, we can make sure we're not supporting child slavery by selecting chocolate from trustworthy sources. Unfortunately, child slavery has been documented even on farms that source chocolate bearing the Fair Trade and Rainforest Alliance certifications.[52] The Food Empowerment Project recommends that consumers not purchase any chocolate coming from West Africa. The other major source of chocolate in the world is Latin America, where there has been no documented slavery in the industry. The Food Empowerment Project also maintains a list of ethical chocolate.[53]

The Coffee Industry

Coffee is another crop associated with a host of ethical issues including exploitation and modern slavery. Child labor is rampant in the coffee industry, and debt slavery is common. The latter is where laborers, many of them children, become indebted to landowners and are forced to repay their debts through what amounts to indentured servitude.

The exploitation of the coffee industry is not limited to human beings either. Until we come to see that other living beings are not born for us to use for our own ends, humanity will continue to discover new ways of exploiting them. Take, for example, Kopi luwak, an Indonesian specialty coffee produced by force-feeding coffee beans to the Asian palm civet, a small mammal found in the rainforests of Asia. Excreted beans are harvested for human consumption. This "civet coffee" has led to intensive farming of the animals, who are confined in battery cages and force-fed the coffee beans.[54] Though it would seem that this practice would remain relatively obscure (given that it involves eating excrement), Kopi luwak has become quite trendy, even being featured on the Oprah Winfrey Show and in the 2007 film *The Bucket List*.

Coffee production is also responsible for devastating environmental degradation, primarily as a result of rejecting traditional methods of growing coffee under the shade of the forest canopy in favor of full sunlight. Shade-grown coffee helps prevent soil erosion and provides habitat for wildlife, but it can be more costly. Thus, many coffee growers opt for the higher-profit yield—clear-cutting forests and destroying habitat and soil quality in the process. This practice doesn't just affect the local wildlife but wildlife throughout the region. For example, hundreds of millions of birds from hundreds of species migrate annually through Central America, where much of the world's coffee is grown.[55] Studies in Colombia and Mexico have identified over ninety percent fewer bird species in sun-grown plantations than in shade coffee.[56] Sun-grown coffee is also more susceptible to pests, and therefore requires more agricultural chemicals and fungicides. Depletion of the soil necessitates more chemical fertilizers, making coffee the third most heavily sprayed crop in the world.[57]

The more aware we are of where our foods come from, the more empowered we are to use our dollars to vote for a more just and sustainable world. But we need to be mindful even when evaluating the certifications, as their value varies widely. Organic certification ensures crops are grown without the damaging pesticides that harm our own health and the environment, but it does not address the issues of human rights. At present, the Rainforest Alliance Certification has such low standards it is hardly meaningful at all. The Fair Trade certification guarantees a fixed price to growers, but with fluctuations in the market price of coffee even this does not mean a living wage. The Food Empowerment Project lists a few truly sustainable coffee companies but advises that finding ethical coffee is so difficult we should aim to reduce or eliminate our coffee consumption entirely. Economic reality is always based on many interrelated factors, and some might argue that boycotting coffee would only further harm growers. So there may not be one simple answer. Our practice is to be mindful, to be open, and to investigate our own attachments to see where they do us or others harm. Then we make our best efforts, with as much information as possible, to make compassionate and wise choices.

Food Deserts

When we understand and can question the realities of food production, we can begin to reform the system. Our current system favors big corporate conglomerates profiting off food that is bad for human health, bad for the animals, and bad for the environment. Access to healthy food highlights racial and economic inequalities in our society. According to the World Health Organization, the right to health is a basic human right: this includes access to health care, clean water, and healthy food.[58] By this definition, many Americans, particularly ethnic minorities and the poor, are being denied this basic human right.

Besides those experiencing actual hunger or food insecurity, an even larger segment of the population live in "food deserts," geopolitical regions "where residents' access to affordable, healthy food options (especially fresh fruits and vegetables) is restricted or nonexistent due to the absence of grocery stores within convenient travelling distance."[59] Studies have found that there are three times as many supermarkets in wealthier areas than in poorer communities, and that predominantly white neighborhoods contain an average of four times as many supermarkets as predominantly black ones do.[60] Conversely, food deserts often have an overabundance of *unhealthy* food, including the meat-and-dairy-based fatty, salty, and sugary foods found in fast food restaurants and convenience stores. Lack of access to healthy foods is one of the main reasons that minority and low-income populations suffer from statistically higher rates of many of the diseases of affluence including obesity, type 2 diabetes, cardiovascular disease, and other diet-related conditions.[61]

Urban agriculture and community gardens offer some hope, since both teach local residents about healthy foods and make them available, usually for no charge at all. Supporting these urban community gardens is one of the best ways to help bring about food justice in the communities most in need of healthy, affordable food.

Purchasing food through Community Supported Agriculture (CSAs) or at farmers markets is another way to support local growers and transform our food system. Buying directly from local growers assures that the foods we buy haven't been transported over long distances, contributing to carbon emissions and greenhouse gases. Buying directly from the farmer also cuts out the middleman, so the grower receives the full profit. When we buy from large grocery stores, much of the price of the produce goes to the store, leaving less for the grower.

Traditional farming methods relied on crop rotation to keep soil healthy, but modern technological advancements and intensified farming methods have encouraged mega-farms, specialized production, crop monocultures, and mechanization—all of which lead to a plethora of environmental problems and undermine good nutrition.[62] Farmers selling through farmers markets and CSAs are more likely to offer greater variety than that found in the large grocery chains, which benefits both the environment and our own personal health.

Palm Oil

Palm oil is grown throughout Africa, Asia, North America, and South America, but eighty-five percent of all palm oil is produced and exported from Indonesia and Malaysia.[63] Indonesian palm oil is linked to destruction of primary forest and habitat destruction for a large number of endangered species including the orangutan and Sumatran tiger. The development of oil palm plantations has forcibly displaced communities of indigenous people.[64]

Palm oil is found in half of the products we buy, from processed foods to personal care products and detergents.[65] This is why environmental groups like Greenpeace believe change will have to come from corporate leadership.[66] Large companies like Pepsi have the power to change the industry, but corporations will only change when consumers use their purchasing power to pressure corporations to do so. In 2008, the Roundtable on Sustainable Palm Oil (RSPO) developed a set of environmental and social criteria with which companies must comply in order to produce Certified Sustainable Palm Oil (CSPO). Criteria include a commitment not to clear primary forest, to reduce pesticide use, and to ensure fair labor practices. By this point, we must have surely become expert label readers, so we can put this important skill to use and add palm oil to the list of ingredients we look for, only purchasing products with the Certified Sustainable Palm Oil trademark.

When we look deeply into our food, where it comes from, the impact on Earth, on the animals, workers, and our own health, we can truly see the interconnection of all things. It's no longer a theory or philosophy with which we agree or disagree; it's simply the truth that we can now see once we've become mindful and honest with ourselves. Once we see this great truth, our choices naturally begin to evolve toward those that lead to greater peace, happiness, and well-being for all. We don't have to fight or force ourselves. Mindfulness helps generate a genuine interest in adopting right diet, which gives us the energy to make changes that bring us a profound peace that only comes from living in harmony with our highest Selves. ✱

3

The Mind–Body Connection

Physical Fitness

Regular exercise is strongly linked with good health. People who exercise regularly have healthier body weights and are at a reduced risk for a range of diseases and illnesses including diabetes, certain cancers, heart disease, and arthritis, among others. Their quality of life is better, and they're more able to fight diseases like cancer if they do occur. People who engage in regular physical activity have more energy and better moods; they sleep better and report having more satisfying sex lives.

Life is good. We all want to live. This is just part of the fabric of existence: the drive to continue life, to stay alive, to propagate more life. We need to stay strong and fit and healthy for our own sake, for our own happiness and peace, but also so we're able to be there for others: from our families (whether that be healthy children or sick parents), to our neighbors, to the limitless number of beings who suffer from every imaginable form of hardship. Good health makes our spiritual practices much easier, and we must be healthy if we are to serve.

Exercise plays an essential role in good health when we engage in it appropriately, meaning in a way and to a degree that promotes health and wellness in all areas of being. True health lies in our ability to synthesize mind, body, and soul, to integrate these parts and see that these are all facets of an indivisible whole. Tending to one facet and not the others is like showering and only washing our upper body, or only brushing our front teeth. No, we want to wash the whole body! We want to brush all the teeth! Similarly, we want to purify, cleanse, and nourish our whole being, which is (at this point in our journeys) an inextricable mixture of elements of body, mind, and soul.

Just like when we drive through rush-hour traffic, we can get caught up in our own impatience and start driving like maniacs: peeling out and burning rubber at every traffic light; cutting people off, blowing our horns, and unleashing all manner of expletives at the old lady who stops in front of us when the light is still yellow. Or we can remain mindful and watch ourselves as we maneuver through the obstacle course of life, staying present and aware of the full range of emotions we feel in all areas of our lives.

We'll see the ego just as we go down into that head-to-knee stretch and feel that pull in the ligament behind the knee. There's a voice of reason that says, "OK, that's far enough," but the ego won't abide what it perceives as weakness. It'll tell us to push further. It'll convince us, crazy as it seems when we can look at the situation rationally, that somehow we'd be a much better person—much worthier, stronger, more attractive, etc.—if we'd just keep pushing. So we push despite a very unpleasant and sharp tension that eventually will go snap, and then you know what that crazy ego will say, right? It'll say, "You idiot! Why are you so stupid? So vain?!" The ego is volatile, unreliable, with unrealistic expectations and never satisfied, though at times inflated with a false and fragile sense of pride.

We can keep the ego in check by paying attention to our thoughts; by learning to differentiate between the thoughts and motives driven by the ego and those driven by the higher egoless consciousness; and by keeping our ultimate goals in mind at all times. So when we walk into the gym and we're paying attention, we may notice the ego as it peers around the corner, waiting to attack. Before it has a chance to run out and start screaming, we can say "I see you!" and draw ourselves back to our center through mindfulness—reminding ourselves that physical fitness is about much more than appearance, which will fade, no matter what we do. Exercise is an essential component of health and well-being: to allow us to pursue our spiritual practices, be around for our children or our grandchildren, and to serve all beings.

There are so many different ways of staying fit. If we can find what feels good and what we enjoy, we're more likely to stick with it. As with creating any habit, it helps to establish a routine. For example, you might create a weekly exercise schedule. Try to exercise at the same time every day so you create a real habit. I have to admit, I hardly ever really feel like brushing my teeth, but I do it every morning when I get up because it's a habit; and I definitely feel better once I've done it! It's the same with exercising (or meditating, or any other habit we're trying to establish).

Exercise guidelines will vary for different individuals and age groups; but generally, most people between the ages of eighteen and sixty-five, with no major health complications (and if you have any health concerns or complications you should speak with a physician before starting a fitness routine), should aim for a minimum of thirty minutes a day, or three and a half hours per week of moderate to vigorous aerobic activity (any activity that raises your heart rate so that you can still talk but with difficulty). This could be jogging outdoors, bicycling, hiking, dancing, or swimming, among other activities.

Aerobic activity probably doesn't include yoga, unless you're engaging in one of the more strenuous forms, such as *Ashtanga* or power *vinyasa*. These styles of yoga are a great workout but can be difficult for many bodies. Even if you are physically fit enough for these styles, some people simply prefer to keep their yoga more meditative and gentler.

In addition to the aerobic activity, we also want to add a couple of days of strength training, working all the major muscle groups of the body (legs, hips, back, chest, abdomen, shoulders, and arms). Strength training might include lifting weights, working with resistance bands, or using your own body weight as resistance (push-ups, sit-ups, or yogasana).

Yogasana and Pranayama (the Physical Postures of Yoga and Breath Control)

In America, for the most part, yoga is associated with yogasana. Asanas are the physical postures of yoga. Yoga is commonly considered a form of exercise, but it isn't that. As Swami Satyananda Saraswati says, yoga consists of "techniques which place the physical body in positions that cultivate awareness, relaxation, concentration and meditation."[1]

Hatha Yoga

We often forget that we are more than our bodies. Much more. But for the time being, we need these bodies. And we need to keep them healthy so we can get on with the joy of being alive and living out our unique purpose on the planet, whatever that might be. *Hatha yoga* refers to the practices compiled in the *Hatha Yoga Pradipika*, written by Swāmi Svātmārāma in the fifteenth century C.E. It is particularly concerned with helping us find health in the physical body as a means to something higher.

Whereas raja yoga begins with ethics, hatha yoga starts with purifying the body through asana, pranayama, and other cleansing practices. The sages who devised hatha yoga believed that the mind needed to be tamed through the physical practices before it would be stable enough to be able to follow the ethics, and then ultimately to master meditation.

The word *hatha* comes from *ha*, representing prana *shakti*, or the life force running through us, and *tha*, representing *manas* shakti, or mental energy. Hatha yoga is the union of these two forces. It is believed that when these two forces come together, we achieve higher states of consciousness. When our energy is blocked either by physical or emotional and mental congestion, illness develops, hindering our ability to function properly in almost every way imaginable: to think, digest, feel, and express ourselves.

According to the science of hatha yoga, three major energy channels, or *nadis*, run along the spine. (The nadis roughly correspond to the meridian points in Chinese medicine. The ancient rishis tell us there are 72,000 of these channels throughout the body.) The channels are something like nerves, but they exist on an energetic level. *Ida* nadi represents the negative flow and equates roughly to *yin* in the Chinese energy system. *Pingala* represents the positive flow and equates to *yang* in the Chinese system. *Sushumna* nadi is the main energy channel that represents the neutral flow of spiritual energy. Ida is said to begin in *muladhara*, the root *chakra* (the energy vortex) located at the base of the spine, and end at the left nostril. Pingala also begins in the root chakra and ends at the right nostril. The two channels intersect like the double helix of our DNA, crossing each other at every chakra. Sushumna also begins in the root chakra, travels directly parallel to the spine, and runs to the top of the head at the crown chakra known as *sahasrara*.

Hatha yoga is primarily concerned with balancing these energies and the union of these three main energy channels at the eyebrow center, otherwise known as the *ajna* or third eye chakra. In this way, physical and mental purification and balance is achieved.

In the *Yoga Sutras*, Patanjali defines *yogasana* as "*sthira sukham asanam*," meaning that posture which is steady and sweet, or comfortable. For the raja yogi, then, asana is primarily the stable seated posture used for meditation. The hatha yogis, however, found that certain physical postures help us open different energy channels and psychic centers, and that controlling the body enables us to control the mind. As such, the physical postures become another tool in the quest for spiritual enlightenment, a means to an end and not an end in themselves.

This distinction may have gotten a little lost in modern America, where we're apt to overemphasize yogasana to the exclusion of the rest of the practices of yoga. But keeping the body supple and fit is an essential part of a contemplative life, whether we want to sit in meditation or focus on any other aspect of our practice or our lives without being distracted or deterred by the aches and pains of a broken-down body.

Yogasana is also beneficial in ways that go beyond preparation for seated meditation. For example, many yoga postures are modeled after animals in nature, reflecting the understanding of the ancient forest-dwelling rishis who lived harmoniously with nature. They watched the animals and believed that if we could model ourselves after them, we also could find more harmony with nature and our own bodies.

I've often had the same idea as I've sat and watched birds of all sizes and colors fluttering about so naturally, without the self-doubt or hesitation we humans so often feel. They don't struggle to understand themselves or their purpose. They just are: authentic and without the neurosis of identity or identity crises. In different asanas, we model ourselves after these animal teachers. For example, according to Swami Satyananda Saraswati, "by imitating the rabbit or hare in *shashankasana*, [we can] . . . influence the flow of adrenaline responsible for the 'fight or flight' mechanism."[2]

Yoga postures generally fall into the following categories: forward bends, backward bends, twists, inversions, standing strength postures, balance postures, and relaxation postures. In forward folds we stretch the muscles of the back and the hamstrings, and on a psychic level we introvert ourselves, tuning out the outside world and looking within. In backbends, we increase flexibility in the spine, which is central to good health. In India, it's a common adage that "you are only as old as your spine." Nerves connect the spine to the limbs and all the major organs of the body. If the spine is inflexible, nerve impulses become blocked, leading to a range of disorders through the body and making us more susceptible to disease. Backbends also help us extrovert ourselves, so we can let go of fear and find confidence.

Through twists, we squeeze out the internal organs, eliminating toxins and improving digestion by stimulating peristalsis, the contraction and relaxation of muscles that help digestion move along. The standing strength postures build muscle and increase both mental and physical strength, while the balance postures help us find our center of gravity and our calm focus. All the postures combined increase flexibility, build immunity, and tone and massage the endocrine glands. According to Sri Swami Satchidananda, "[w]ith proper diet and proper Yoga practices, asanas, and breathing, one can overcome almost all types of diseases."[3]

Yoga also helps us understand that for every mental knot we have—every neurosis, every bit of tension—we have a corresponding knot or point of tension in the body. That's part of being human. Whether I fight with my partner over whose turn it is to take out the trash, or a dog runs out in front of me and I have to swerve my car into a ditch to avoid hitting him, my body will tense up in response to stress, especially the muscles in what's called the "tension triangle."

The tension triangle is formed by the shoulders at the base and forehead at the peak. When we experience stress, we engage muscles in this zone most notably. We furrow our brows, clench our jaws, grind our teeth, hunch our shoulders, and tighten our necks. This is part of the fight-or-flight mechanism. Our bodies are evolutionarily designed to manifest psychological stress as muscle tension, among other processes.

The functions of the body that happen automatically and that we cannot usually control by will are regulated by the body's autonomic nervous system, which is further divided into the sympathetic and the parasympathetic nervous systems. The sympathetic nervous system is triggered in stressful situations: the fight-or-flight mode. The parasympathetic nervous system is triggered when the mind and body are at rest and is known as rest-and-digest mode.

In its way, stress is the body's biological alarm that sounds when we feel threatened. In emergency situations, our fight-or-flight response can save our lives. When we're stressed, the brain sets off a combination of nerve and hormonal signals that prompt the adrenal glands to release a surge of hormones, including adrenaline and cortisol. Adrenaline raises the heart rate, elevates blood pressure, and boosts energy supplies. Cortisol inflates sugars in the bloodstream, enhances our brain's use of glucose, and increases the availability of substances that repair tissues. This symphony of biological changes helps prepare us to respond quickly to the threat. Cortisol also turns off certain functions that would hinder our ability to react to emergency situations, like the immune and digestive systems.

But in modern life, where daily responsibilities and situations like work, traffic, health problems, separation from family, etc. produce ongoing stress, we get "stuck" in that fight-or-flight mode, and our bodies aren't designed to handle that. We're biologically programmed to respond in the same way to attacking tigers as we are to crying babies, bad drivers, and chemistry tests. Prolonged, daily, low-grade stress tears down the body in many ways. Staying in that fight-or-flight mode can disrupt almost all of our body's processes and put us at risk of heart disease, sleep problems, digestive problems, depression, and obesity.

Pranayama

The breath is often considered the bridge between the mind and the body. Breathing is normally an automatic function of the body. We do it without thinking. That's why we don't die when we take a nap. But breathing is one of the few functions of the body we can control through the mind.

The fourth of Patanjali's eight-limbed system of yoga is *pranayama*, usually referred to as breath control. It is that, but it's also more than that. *Prana* means both "breath" and "life" in Sanskrit. Breath is life. Besides the physical breath, prana also signifies the life force. On a more subtle level than breath control, pranayama has to do with controlling the life force as it flows through the nadis of the body. Poor diet, mental or emotional stress, and irregularities in lifestyle can all deplete or block the pranic flow, leading people to feel drained and to become susceptible to illness and depression. The pranayama, or breathing practices, release these blocks and help us balance prana and revitalize our energy.

Modern science has its own explanation of how this works. Through controlling the breath, we begin to regulate the mind, and as we do this, we control the body. By slowing and deepening the breath, we basically tell the body there is no threat, and that it can switch from fight-or-flight to rest-and-digest. In other words, through deep conscious breathing, we can influence a range of autonomic functions of the body—processes like heart rate, blood pressure, and hormone production—over which we normally have no control. This is why it's so important to begin every yoga practice with conscious deep breathing. As soon as we do, we immediately bring our bodies into the parasympathetic system, where we begin the process of healing and repairing. Of course, we don't have to wait for a yoga class to begin breathing.

Basic Mindful Breathing

Find your comfortable seat. Close your eyes and observe the breath. Notice as it naturally begins to slow and deepen. Begin to count the breath in the following manner: Inhale, one. Exhale, two. Inhale, three. Exhale, four. Continue until you reach ten. Then reverse-count back to one. If you lose count or become distracted, begin again.

We incorporate pranayama into our hatha practice by staying mindful of the breath through the practice. I practiced "yoga" for about eight years without knowing there was any connection between yoga and breathing. I learned from my first yoga

Body Scan Breathing Exercise

This is a very simple breathing technique we can use anytime we're feeling stressed, or at the beginning of a hatha yoga practice. It would also be a wonderful practice to include in a daily routine: maybe five minutes in the morning and five minutes before bed.

- If you're at home, find a quiet place and begin in a comfortable seated posture. Sit upright, but be comfortable (so maybe slide a pillow or blanket under your hips). If you're driving or at work, try to do this where you are.
- Stop. Find your breath, and begin to deepen the breath.
- If possible (i.e., you're not in traffic!) close your eyes.
- Breathe into the belly, then draw the breath into the middle chest, then the upper chest. Find a smooth flow of breath. As you exhale, deflate the upper chest, middle chest, and belly.
- Begin to become aware of how the body feels. Notice where you are holding tension through the body. Scan the hips, the belly, the shoulders, the jaw, the face, and the temples, and focus on releasing and softening in those areas.
- Notice if there are thoughts clinging in the mind. Become aware of them, and then try to step back and watch the thought, creating distance between yourself and it, and then bring your awareness back to the breath, noticing and resting in the quiet gaps in between the thoughts.

Nadi Shodhan: Alternate-Nostril Breathing

Another basic pranayama, *nadi shodhan*, or alternate-nostril breathing, helps still the mind while balancing our life-force energies, bringing balance and calm to the mind.

Come to a comfortable seated posture with an upright spine. Relax your whole body and close your eyes. Rest your left hand on your left knee, either with the palm turned upward in a receiving position or in any *mudra* (symbolic gesture) you like, such as *jnana* (wisdom) mudra (the tips of the thumb and forefinger gently touching).

Fold the first and second fingers of the right hand into the palm. Bring your right hand to your face so you can alternately use the right thumb to block the right nostril and the right ring finger to block the left nostril.

Begin by inhaling through both nostrils. Then close your right nostril with your right thumb and exhale completely through your left nostril. Inhale completely though the same nostril. At the end of your inhalation, close off the left nostril with your ring finger and exhale through the right nostril. Inhale through the right nostril and then close the right nostril with the right thumb as you exhale through the left nostril, continuing to alternate the breathing in this way.

Try to maintain a steady, even, and slow breath throughout the practice. Initially, try to inhale for a count of five and exhale for a count of five. Practice for five to ten rounds in this manner, and maintain the inhalation and exhalation at a one-to-one ratio. As you become more comfortable with the practice, you can increase the duration of the breath to a count of ten on both the inhalation and the exhalation, maintaining the one-to-one ratio.

After perfecting this technique, the ratio may be changed to one-to-two, beginning by returning to a five-count on the inhalation and maintaining a ten-count on the exhalation. Increase the duration only when you can practice like this without any strain of any kind.

Heart Breathing Technique

After a few minutes of deep conscious breathing as described above (p. 94), draw the breath up into the heart and feel the sensations there—even if initially you sense there's something there you don't want to feel. Allow yourself to feel fully, and then again come back to the breath and exhale the feelings out. Allow these feelings to wash over you in waves, noticing as they come and as they go.

Breathe in and out of the heart, allowing it to become more tender with each breath. Stay connected to that softness, beyond ego, beyond thought. Find that sweet spot in the center of the heart and let that fill you. Know that is the true Self.

Whenever the mind wanders, try to gently draw yourself back to the breath, to the quiet spaces in between the thoughts. Keep relaxing any part of the body, mind, or heart that tenses back up. Keep coming back to the breath, to the eternal peace at your core that is always there at the center of the ups and downs.

Ujjayi Pranayama

While breathing in and out of the nose, gently close the back of the throat (the glottis) just slightly so that you can hear a soft snoring sound forming at the back of the throat. Because of this sound, the *ujjayi* breath is sometimes called the ocean breath, or the Darth Vader breath! It can help us stay focused on our breathing. It soothes the nervous system, helps us connect to our strength, and calms the mind.

teacher in India that if we aren't controlling the breath, we aren't practicing yoga. When we bring the breath under control, we bring the mind under control. As Patanjali says, *yoga chitta vritti nirodha*, "yoga is the control of the mind."

As we move in and out of physical postures of yoga, we mindfully move the awareness through the body seeking out those knots of tension, and releasing them through a combination of physical and mental practices. We stretch muscles and deepen our breathing to bring more oxygen to various muscles and organs. We invert ourselves to increase blood flow to parts of the body that don't normally receive much blood. We twist to flush out organs. And throughout the entire sequence of postures, we maintain the mind–body connection through the breath.

Different yoga schools emphasize different styles and intensity of asana. In order to benefit the most from a hatha yoga practice, you want to choose a style that best suits your individual needs. As I indicated earlier, if you're young and fit, then you should engage in intense (though safe) forms of exercise, and a style like Ashtanga with its profusely sweaty, fairly grueling, and gymnastic series of postures may be just right for you. But if that sounds a bit much, you can still derive tremendous benefit from a slightly more gentle form of yoga, such as the basic hatha sequence offered below.

Basic Yogasana Sequence for Purity and Longevity

Before beginning this sequence, take a moment to practice the basic breathing exercise outlined above and set an intention for your practice. Through yoga, we seek to release the ego and purify ourselves so we may be of better service to others. Take a moment to dedicate yourself to someone or something other than the ego.

As you go through the sequence, make sure to stay conscious of your breathing. Synchronize the breath with the motion. Keep your eyes closed as much as you can, and try using the ujjayi pranayama so the sound of your breath fills the mind. Throughout our hatha practice, we want to try to breathe in and out of the nose, unless we're congested, or have any other breathing problems.

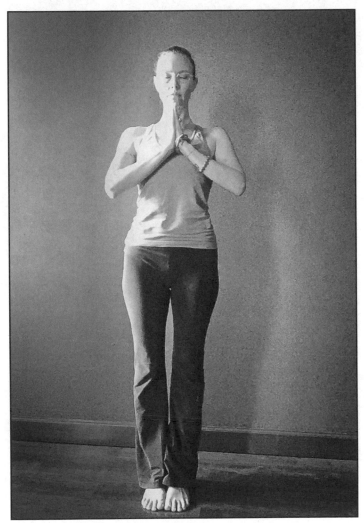

Tadasana
(Mountain)

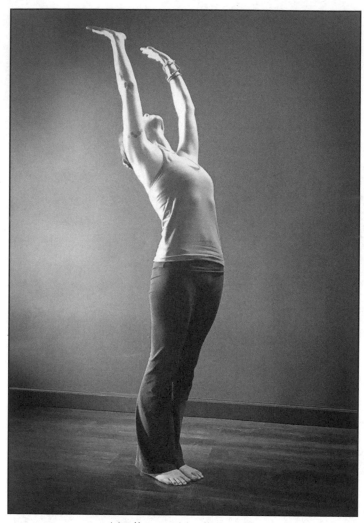

Urdhava Hastasana
(Upward Salute)

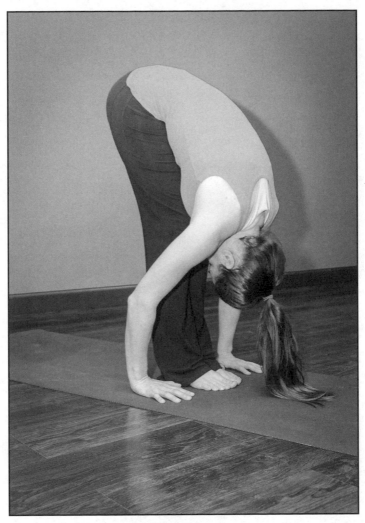

Uttanasana
(Standing Forward Fold)

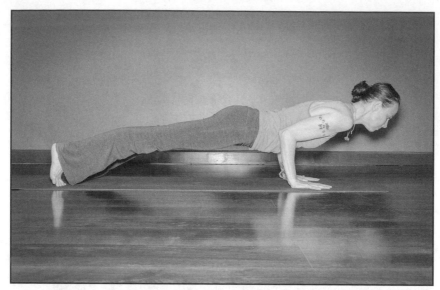

Chaturanga Dandasana
(Four-Limbed Staff)

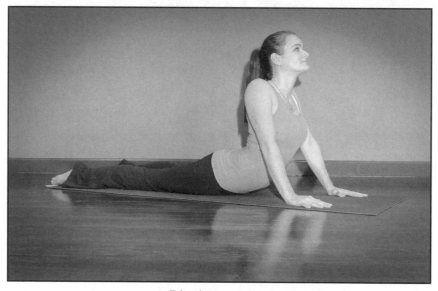

Bhujangasana
(Cobra)

102

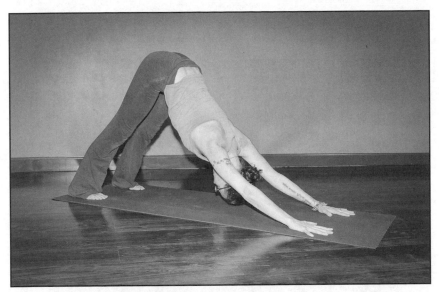

Adho Mukha Svanasana
(Downward-Facing Dog)

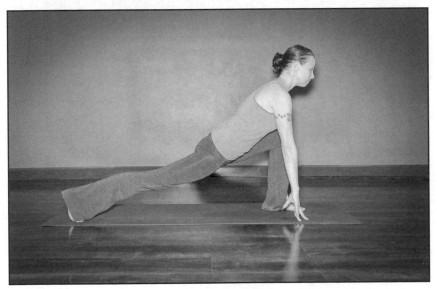

Ashwa Sanchalanasana
(Low Lunge)

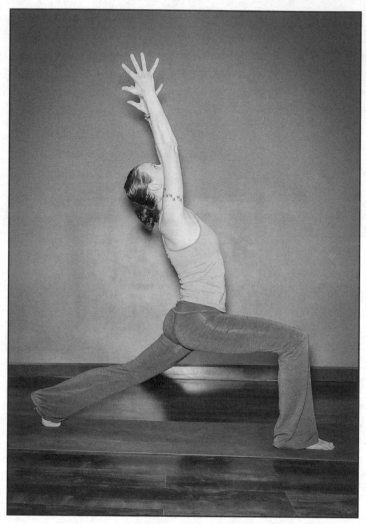

Alanasana
(Crescent Pose High Lunge)

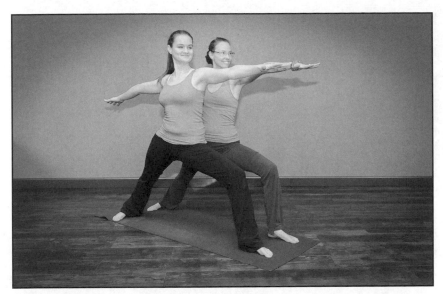

Virabhadrasana 2
(Warrior 2)

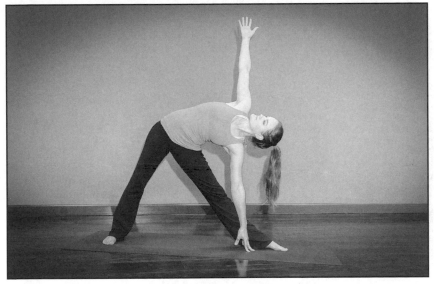

Trikonasana
(Triangle)

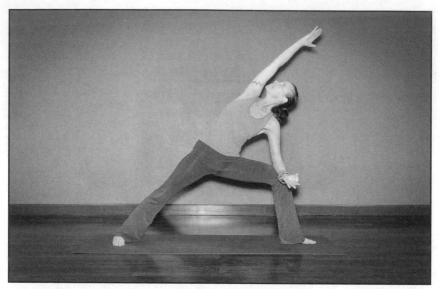

Utthita Parsvakonasana
(Extended Side Angle)

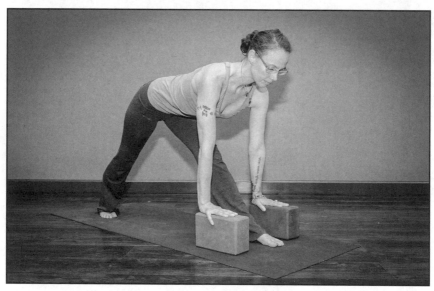

Parsvottanasana
(Intense Side Stretch)

106

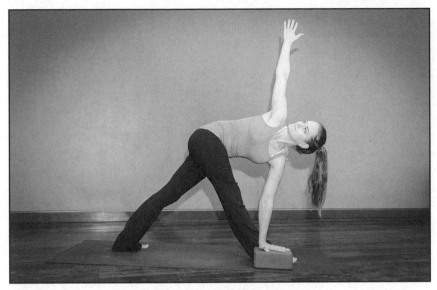

Parivritta Trikonasana
(Revolved Triangle)

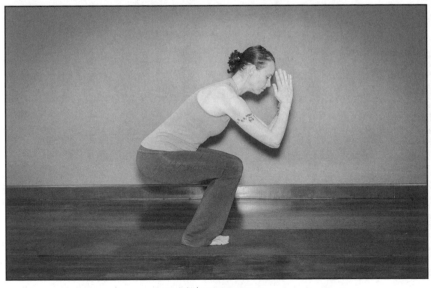

Utkatasana
(Chair Pose—Variation)

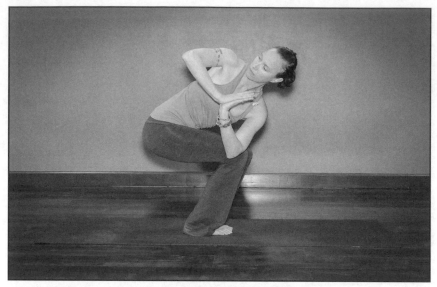

Parivrtta Utkatasana
(Revolved or Twisted Chair)

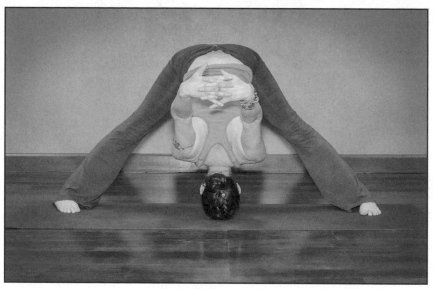

Prasarita Padottanasana
(Wide-legged Forward Bend)

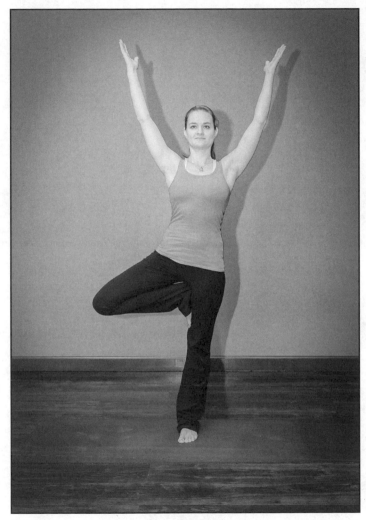

Vrksasana
(Tree)

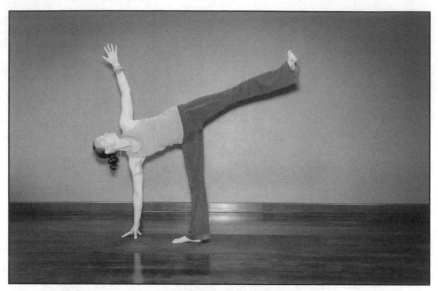

Ardha Chandrasana
(Half Moon)

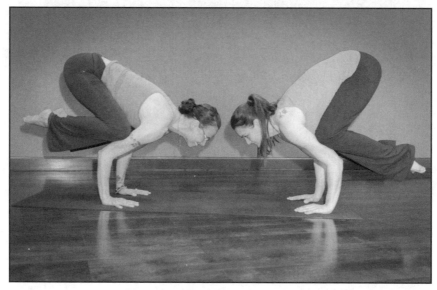

Bakasana
(Crow)

110

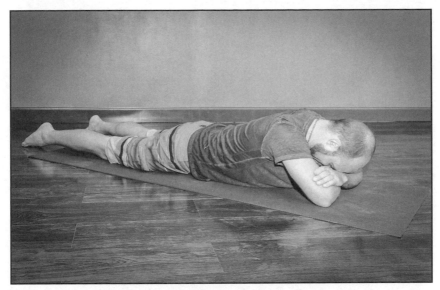

Makarasana
(Crocodile)

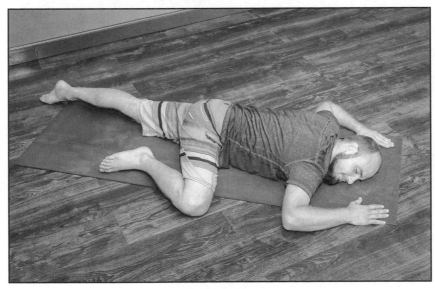

Matsya Kridasana
(Flapping Fish)

111

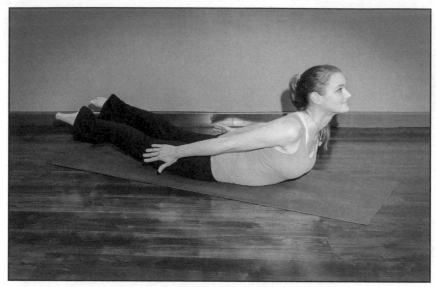

Shalabasana
(Locust)

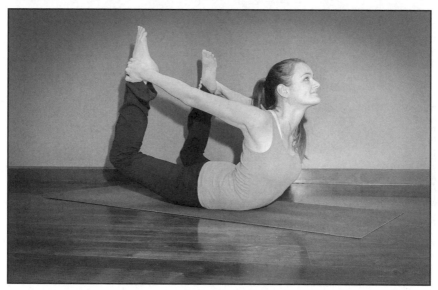

Dhanurasana
(Bow)

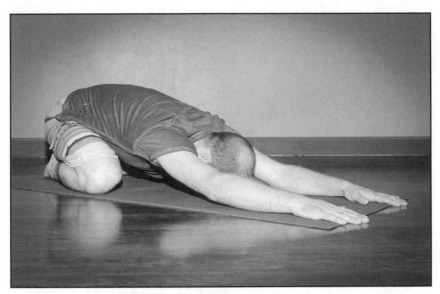

Balasana
(Child)

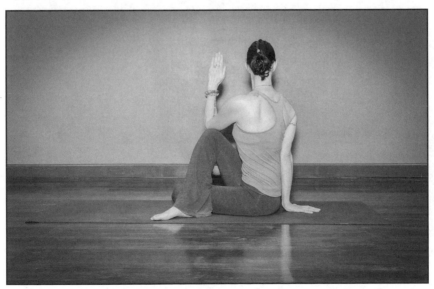

Ardha Matsyendrasana
(Half Spinal Twist)

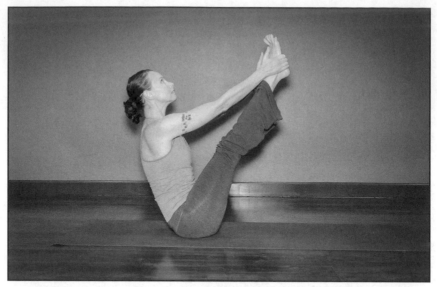

Navasana
(Boat)

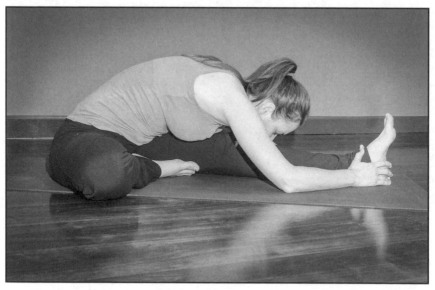

Janu Sirsasana
(Head to Knee)

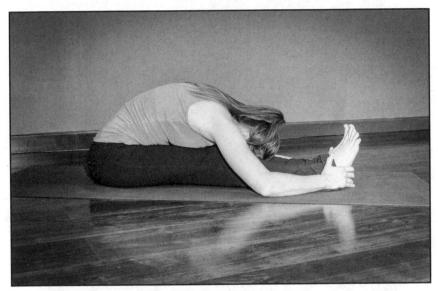

Paschimottanasana
(Seated Forward Bend)

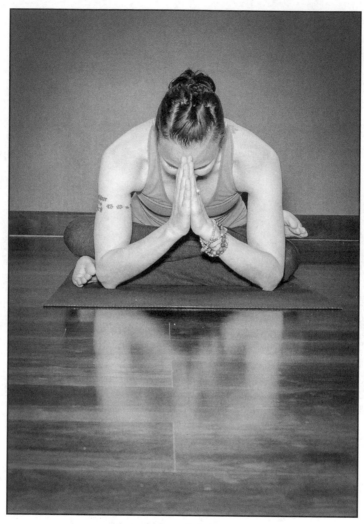

Agnistambhasana
(Fire Log)

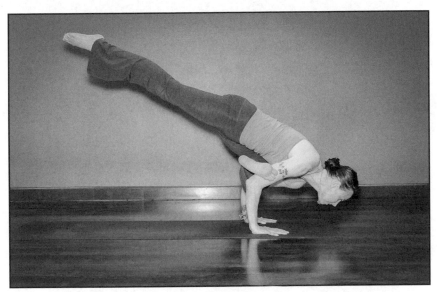

Eka Pada Galavasana
(Flying Pigeon)

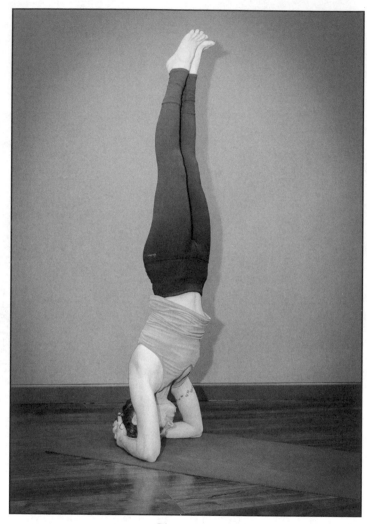

Sirasana
(Headstand)

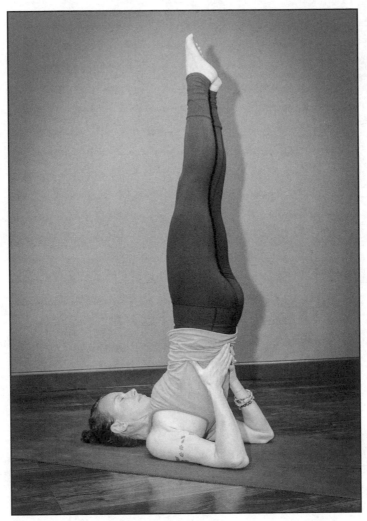

Sarvangasana
(Shoulderstand)

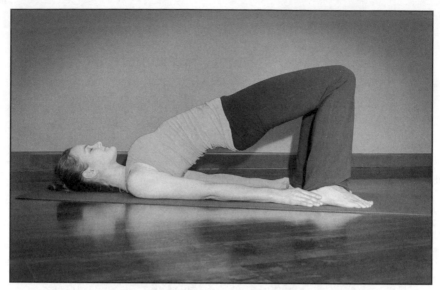

Setu Bandha Sarvangasana
(Bridge)

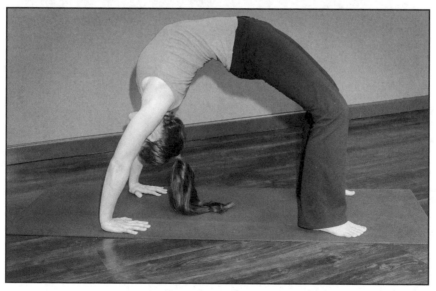

Urdhva Dhanurasana
(Wheel)

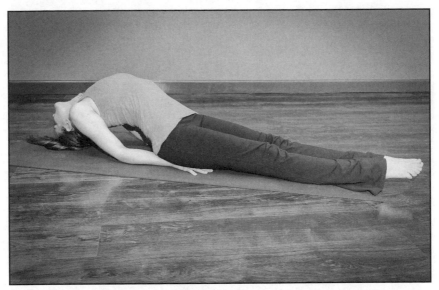

Matsyasana
(Fish)

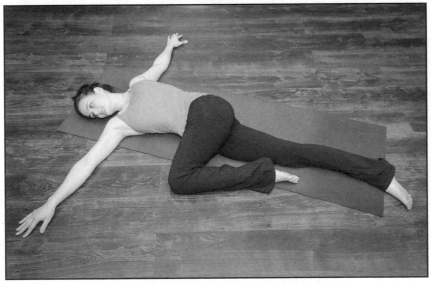

Supta Matsyendrasana
(Supine Spinal Twist)

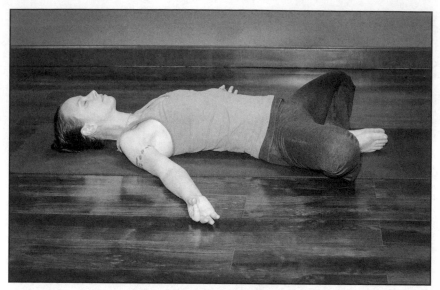

Supta Baddha Konasana
(Reclined Bound Angle)

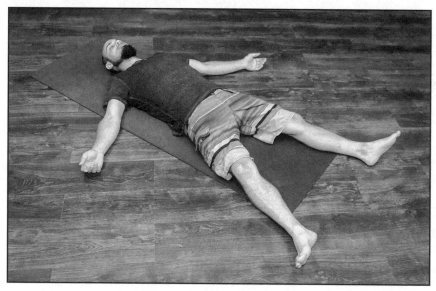

Savasana
(Corpse)

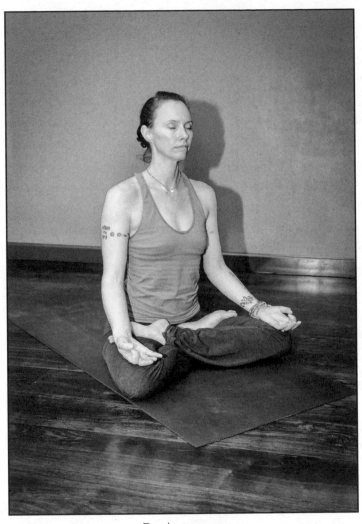

Padmasana
(Lotus)

Additional Advanced Postures: *Virabhadrasana 3* (Warrior 3), *Sirsasana 2* (Tripod Headstand), *Eka Pada Koundinyasana* (Sage Balance)

Kriyas

According to hatha yoga, there are six main cleansing practices that can help us clear energy blocks through the body and balance our energies in order to ascend to higher states of consciousness. These are known as *shatkarma*. *Shat* means "six," and in this context, *karma* means "cleaning." So, we have six main purification or cleansing systems: "Dhauti, basti, neti, trataka, nauli and kapalbhati; these are known as shatkarma (or six cleansing processes)."[4] The aim of the shatkarmas is to create harmony between the two major energetic flows working in the body.

The *Hatha Yoga Pradipika* warns that these practices are so powerful they can be dangerous if practiced improperly and therefore may only be taught directly by a *guru* (realized being) or by someone who has learned them directly from the guru. Therefore, I include them here primarily as reference. Those with the inclination are advised to pursue these further under the guidance and instruction of an experienced teacher. The six shatkarmas are as follows:

Neti: A process of cleansing and purifying the nasal passages

Dhauti (internal cleaning): A series of cleaning in the three main groups: *anthar dhauti*, or internal cleaning; *sirha dhauti*, or head cleaning (traditionally called *dantha dhauti*); and *hrid dhauti*, or thoracic cleaning

Nauli: A method of massaging and strengthening the abdominal organs

Basti: Techniques for washing and toning the large intestine

Kapalbhati: A breathing technique for purifying the frontal region of the brain

Trataka: The practice of intense gazing at one point or object, which develops the power of concentration ❀

4

Cleansing the Soul

We can clean our skin with soap. We can purify our insides by eating pure food, drinking pure water, sweating, wringing out the organs with asana, and exhaling toxins with deep cleansing breathing, but how do we clean our hearts and our souls? It's kind of a trick question, because yoga teaches us that we don't need to clean the heart and soul. They are always pure, eternally unsullied by this world. Our work lies not in purging the soul, but in reconnecting with it. The practice is to cast off all the many layers of ignorance and attachment, of fear and ego, that cloak the Divine Self within our hearts. Our task is to surrender to the love within ourselves that will cleanse and heal all of our wounds. Love will wash away all the dirt and grime that may seem to be a part of our DNA, but which yoga teaches us is just part of the illusion, just temporary layers of skin waiting to be shed.

* * *

When I was first laid off from the law firm, I felt an enormous sense of relief. But after about six months, I was just about out of money and still hadn't figured out what to do with my life. The situation with my fiancé had only gotten worse, as his disease progressed along with my codependency. I had very limited emotional resources for dealing with what had begun to feel like a full-blown life crisis, and

125

I was consumed by my own personal suffering. I was anxiety-ridden, insecure, and filled with jealousy, not to mention self-doubt and despair.

I would attend one yoga class a week, and during that hour I felt some peace and wholeness. I felt anchored and sensed some amount of hope. I knew that when I was practicing I was able to find peace. But I didn't have the discipline to create a full-time habit. The one hour a week certainly wasn't enough to transform my life, but those glimpses told me that if I had a regular practice, I might be able to do just that.

So I put all of my things in storage, maxed out my credit cards again (having paid them off while at the firm) in order to send my fiancé to drug rehab, drove my animals to Alabama to stay with my father, and with the last of my severance pay flew to India, where I stayed for about two months studying yoga and meditation and discovering a peace I don't think I'd ever known before.

One of the things that happened to me while I was there was that I began exchanging my own personal suffering for that of the world's. I started to let go of my own private dramas and began to see the world again. Every morning at four A.M. I would wake in the darkness and hear the bells clanging around the mules' necks as they started their long workday. Later, in the daylight, I could see the open sores on their hips from where the saddles had rubbed against bone under the weight of the heavy loads they were forced to carry. The men who drove the animals through the narrow alleys of the town were stern-faced and hard-hearted; never in two months did I see a smile soften their pinched faces.

When I went to the sitar lessons I took after yoga class in the afternoons, I passed rows of beggars, many severely disabled, lining the streets, holding out dirty cups for change. I watched as angry men beat hungry cows who tried to steal mangos from their carts. Street dogs were everywhere—skinny, mangy, and hungry and all of them heartbreaking and sweet. There was one dog who hung around outside the gates of the yoga school with whom I fell in love immediately and to whom I would sneak food after meals. One day she wasn't there. And then the next, and the next. I asked the woman who owned the little shop next to the school if she knew where the dog had gone. "To the market," was all she said with a dismissive wave of her hand. "Gone to the market."

The market was a chaotic, bustling, cacophonous area of town filled with shops and cars and flamboyantly colored rickshaws. Although I visited the market many times, I never saw that little dog again. But I started feeding the other skinny little dog who was left behind. Soon she started waiting for me outside the gate of my guesthouse in the dark hours of the early morning, when I'd come out to go to morning yoga practice and feed her the treats I'd bought especially for her. When I'd enter the courtyard of the school, she'd wait outside the gate and play with her friends, other street dogs and the male calves who wandered aimlessly through the labyrinthine alleys of the neighborhood and who fed at the dump across from the school.

Soon the little dog was following me up the stairs to the yoga hall where we had our morning hatha practice. She'd sit outside the door among all the students' shoes and watch the class as we chanted and twisted ourselves up. We opened and closed all of our classes chanting *Om shanti, shanti, shanti*, which is a prayer for peace for all beings. I began thinking of the little dog when I chanted, wishing her peace and using that feeling as a springboard to expand my heart and my wish for peace for all beings. I began calling the little dog Shanti, and soon all the young Indian boys who worked at the school and all of the other Western students said they started thinking of Shanti, too, when they chanted *Om shanti*.

I was keenly tuned in to the suffering around me. Yet, I also felt peace growing and gaining strength within me. My own problems didn't consume me the way they had before. Whenever I chanted *shanti*, I was filled with loving kindness for my loved ones, for that little dog, and for those poor mules with their festering sores. In time, I even began to pray for peace for those seemingly heartless men who whipped and beat the mules as they struggled not to collapse under their unbearably heavy loads. My anger at the abusive men metamorphosed into a genuine wish for their peace, as I came to see the truth that if they experienced peace in their hearts, they'd no longer do harm to those poor animals.

My prayers for their peace may or may not have had any effect on the men, but they did affect me. I changed. Martin Luther King Jr. said, "Darkness cannot drive out darkness; only light can do that. Hate cannot drive out hate; only love can do that."[1] I don't know how much he studied the teachings of the Buddha, but there is a remarkably similar idea found in the *Dhammapada*, where it says, "For hatred can never put an end to hatred; love alone can. This is an unalterable law."[2] It is that love alone that can purify and cleanse the soul.

Are We Ready Now? *Atha Yoga-Anuśāsanam*

Patanjali's *Yoga Sutras* begins with this simple statement: *atha yoga-anuśāsanam*, "Now, therefore, yoga." It's such a Spartan phrase. It's easy to overlook. But this is the way the sutras are written. The teachings were originally passed down orally, so they had to be easy to remember. Yet each word is loaded with a meaning that has to be unpacked, traditionally with the help of a guru or teacher.

The very first word of the sutras is *atha*, which means "now." It implies that we have arrived at a place where we are ready to begin the study and practice of yoga. It implies that something has come before to prepare us for this practice. What this is will be different for everyone. Something has brought us all here, to this place we are—right now—searching for deeper meaning, for more happiness, more peace, better health. Something has prepared us to take this next step.

Although many people wander into their first yoga class with no idea that yoga is more than the physical postures, yoga or any spiritual path is ultimately this search for something more. Converts to any religion are more enthusiastic than those born into a faith. This is true because they've *chosen* their faith. Those of us who adopt or choose a yogic, Buddhist, or any other path have a spirit of real yearning and active volition.

Many of us begin by dabbling. We pick up yoga or Buddhism or tai chi or whatever it is for a while. We feel great while we do it; our lives begin to change. Then we go on vacation, or maybe get sick, or something else happens that throws us off our routine. Suddenly, months or even years have gone by since we practiced. Eventually, we return to the practice and again we feel like we've come home. We know this is what we need to do to stay connected to that peace that is always deep within. But the pattern recycles, and we can bounce back and forth like this for years. Yoga teaches us that we won't really see progress until we practice sincerely, wholeheartedly, and without these breaks.[3]

I also know many people who are drawn to a spiritual path early on, without any sense of pathos driving them. A Vietnamese Buddhist nun I met at Magnolia Grove Monastery in Batesville, Mississippi, Sister Carol, was ordained at the age of thirteen. She is now in her late twenties—the embodiment of purity as well as outright joy. She is as playful as she is wise. She knew even as a child that this was the path she wanted to take. Who knows why some people are able to adopt the practices with such ease, while some of us aren't able to fully surrender until we've reached some level of desperation? For many of us, desperation is a great catalyst for surrender. Whether it's personal tragedy or despair at the state of the world, when we're broken or unfulfilled by the material world we become inclined to turn toward the spiritual.

Of course, we don't have to travel to India or anywhere else to surrender. We find our peace within or we don't find it at all. It can happen anywhere. As long as we're chasing it outside, we won't find it; or if we do, it won't last.

Personally, I experienced peace for the first time in India, but then I had to come home. When I did, it was a pretty big shock to my system. I came back feeling like the Buddha. Then I had my first reunion with my fiancé. Within hours, I felt like I'd lost everything I thought I'd gained during those magical months in India. My sense of victimhood, anger, and jealousy returned with a vengeance. Before we finally ended things, our fights were at least as caustic as they'd been before I left. I felt like a terrible failure.

Then I began the hard work of applying the teachings to my daily life, to these challenges that were a part of it. I hadn't gone to India to run away or with the delusion that my trip would fix everything. I went because I wanted help creating habits that I'd be able to use back home. In the *Bhagavad Gita*, Krishna tells Arjuna to devote himself to "the disciplines of yoga, for yoga is skill in action." (2:50). Yoga gives us the tools we need to live in the world while remaining connected to the Divine Self. Yoga offers us skillful means so we can stay engaged and active in life while maintaining our peace. It's not just a theory; it's a practice.

Samadhi Pada—Portion on Practice

Patanjali's *Yoga Sutras* provides us with a range of practices to develop these skillful means. My own copy is well worn. In the very first sutra of the second book, which is the portion on the practice (in contrast to the theory) of yoga, Patanjali says the practice of yoga is comprised of *tapas, svadhyaya,* and *ishvara pranidhana.*

Tapas literally means "to burn or generate heat." It is the practice of self-discipline or learning to restrain the mind, body, and senses. There are three types of austerities: first, austerity of the physical body; second, austerity of communication and speech; and, third, austerity of the mind.

All mystical traditions share this idea that we must cleanse and purify ourselves to be closer to God. For many yogis and other mystics, tapas, or self-discipline, has led to severe self-denial. From St. Simeon the Stylite, the Syriac ascetic saint who lived on a pillar for over thirty years, to India's standing *babas,* who seek enlightenment through a vow not to sit or lie down (even to sleep) for at least twelve years, austerity has often meant self-torture. Of this kind of self-harm, Lord Krishna says, "Some invent harsh penances. Motivated by hypocrisy and egotism, they torture their innocent bodies and me who dwells within (17:5–6)."

After spending several years as an ascetic himself, the Buddha also rejected extreme forms of self-deprivation. Once, when he could see that one of his monks had overexerted himself in his practices, he reminded him of his days as a sitar player. If we tune the strings so they're too tight, he told him, they'll break. If we tune them so they're too loose, they fall off and make no sound at all. In order to play beautiful music, the Buddha said, we need to tune the strings so they're neither too tight nor too loose. This is the Buddha's Middle Path. This is the path of self-discipline.[4]

Tapas is a burning desire for enlightenment, an all-consuming yearning for purification that gives us the strength of will to actually implement those practices that help us release ego and uncover the Spirit within. This is what it takes for us to make the sometimes hard but necessary decisions to create the lives we want. Enlightenment or *moksha* (liberation) won't come to those of us who are half-hearted or cling to our egos or the pleasures of the senses. Moksha comes to those who burn for truth at the core of our being. Tapas is the fire that burns within us and burns away ego and *samskaras* (deep unconscious mental impressions that create habit energies, discussed further below); it gives us the strength and courage to discipline ourselves, with compassion; to follow the yamas and the niyamas; and to control our bodies, minds, and senses. We are what we think; we become what we put our attention into. We purify ourselves through the heat of our practice.

Svadhyaya is the study of the Divine Self. Traditionally, this is thought to be done through scriptural study. But svadhyaya also includes any practices that help us to know the Divine Self, or Atman. Above all, we must experience the Self for ourselves. When we read scripture or study with a guru or other qualified teacher, we reconnect to a wisdom we've always had within. When we read the *Gita* or *Upanishads*, we aren't reading in order to learn something new, but to awaken a deep knowledge and wisdom that's been forgotten. Swami Satchidananda said, "God cannot be understood by books alone . . . nothing can equal experience."[5] Svadhyaya is not just intellectual study. We may be an expert on the *Gita*, but if we don't know its truth in our soul, we haven't understood it and we don't know the Self. True yoga happens beyond the mind. When we apply tapas to svadhyaya, we discover the necessity of the third component of practice as defined by Patanjali: ishvara pranidhana, total surrender to the Divine.

To surrender in yoga is certainly not to give up. It is to surrender to the goodness in our own hearts, to Divine consciousness. In Christian terms, it is the movement that brings us to the exclamation, "Lord, not by my will, but by thy will be done" (Luke 22:42). It implies the total release of ego-clinging and a willingness to dedicate the fruits of our actions to the Divine. Swami Satchidananda says it is to dedicate the fruits of our actions to "God in manifestation." What is God in manifestation? The German mystic Meister Eckhart said, "Every creature is a word of God."[6] So surrendering to the Divine, the God in manifestation, is therefore to surrender ourselves to all beings, to serve all beings, and dedicate ourselves to the welfare of humanity, animals, trees: the whole of life. It is to live in the spirit of this beautiful mantra:

Lokah Samastha Sukinoh Bhavantu
May all beings everywhere be happy and free, and may the thoughts, words, and actions of my own life contribute in some way to that happiness and to that freedom for all.[7]

The Path to Enlightenment

"Enlightenment" is such a big scary word. It sounds like something reserved for some ethereal being in monastic robes, head freshly shaven, androgynous and foreign, and from an altogether distant time and place—in fact, more for mythological characters than for real people of any age. But what is enlightenment, really? According to the Buddha, it's simply waking up. There's a famous story about the Buddha's encounter with a *brahmin* (priest). The story goes that one day this priest passed the Buddha on the road. As he did, he was struck by the Buddha's radiance and aura of peace. So he stopped the Buddha and asked, "Are you a celestial being or a god?"

"No," said the Buddha.

"Well, then, are you some kind of magician or wizard?"

Again the Buddha answered, "No."

Stumped, the brahmin finally asked, "Well then, what *are* you?" To which the Buddha simply replied, "I am awake."

When we pause to consider this observation we might begin to understand how much we sleepwalk through our lives. What does it mean to be *awake*? When we emerge from our dreams in the morning, do we really wake up or do we just enter another layer of sleep? When we open our eyes, do we look at our partner or our cat with eyes of love and appreciation or do we groan and brace ourselves for the day?

I remember taking the trash out one unremarkable night and noticing the sky was the most extraordinary shade of azure. I paused to absorb it, as the color grew richer and glowed almost golden. I wanted to bathe in it and drink it in; it was so deliciously pleasing to my senses. It occurred to me that the sky was likely this same shade quite often, or maybe not; but its changes were certainly worth noting, though I'd usually been too distracted to notice. Since that moment, rarely a day or night has gone by that I haven't tried to pay attention to the ever-changing and breathtaking light show in the sky surrounding our planet.

How many layers of awakening are there? When we take that first step outside each day, do we inhale and smell the fragrant flowers in bloom? Do we hear the complex, lyrical songs of all the different bird species living in the trees surrounding our house? These are our neighbors. Imagine if we were equally oblivious to the people in the house next door. When we're running to our cars at lunch, do we see the tiny purple flowers growing between the cracks of the broken pavement at the edge of the parking lot? How often do we take a deep breath and remember how fragile and miraculous our lives are—how, at any moment, they could be cut off? Remember we're living on a truly extraordinary planet in a vast universe; that our bodies are made of recycled stardust. This is waking up. That's all enlightenment is. At first, we catch glimpses of such awareness, and eventually these moments of clarity form an unbroken chain.

In many Buddhist practice centers, a bell is rung every so often to wake up the monks and nuns—not because they're actually sleeping, like lying in a heap on the floor, but because their minds, like ours, simply wander away from the miracle of the present moment. Even if we don't live in monastic communities, with a bit of discipline and an interest in awakening we can use all of the sounds that surround us to wake ourselves up.

When we meditate in the mornings, we can allow the birds outside the window to serve as our mindfulness bell. When our minds stray to the list of things we have to do or the discomfort we still feel at the thought of a past experience, the blue jay calling his mate from a nearby branch or the quiet snore of the cat sleeping by our side can call us back to the present. Thich Nhat Hanh says, "When I hear a bird sing, if I return deeply to myself and breathe and smile, that bird reveals the

Buddha's . . . [teaching]. People who are awake can hear the . . . [teaching] being preached in a pebble, a bamboo, or the cry of a baby. . . ."[8]

Awakening and enlightenment are available to us. That is the message of all the truly great spiritual teachers. We can wake up right now no matter what we've done, or what has been done to us; or if we've done nothing, or nothing has been done to us. The message we receive from the people who've woken up, those who've found peace and freedom, who've transcended fear and discovered unconditional love for all in their hearts, is that we are all Divine. We often call these teachers "sages" or "Buddhas," or give them some other such title that makes them seem different from us when in fact what they're calling out is that they're *not* different. We just need to wake up to see it. It's not that I am special, or you are special . . . or maybe I am and you are, too, and so is everyone else—from the tiny little tree frog peeping out in back of the house on those balmy summer nights, to the twelve-year-old girl in the refugee camp in East Africa, to the quiet coworker in the cubicle next to us.

Stories of Redemption

Though most of us have the self-effacing habit of viewing the sages, Buddhas, saints, and other great teachers as inherently different from us, if we look at their own biographies and other sacred scriptural stories, we see that it's often their own flaws and humanity, so much like our own, that's led to their awakening. It's often the darkness itself that spurs us to search for light. We see that, in truth, we are not different from these great souls.

The Prodigal Son

The prodigal son is the classic story of the bad boy who seeks redemption. As told in the Christian Bible, the younger of two sons asks his kindhearted father to split the family's estate prematurely so he can take an early inheritance. The father consents, and the young son takes off, quickly squandering his wealth on "wild living" (Luke 15:11–32: New International Version). When he finds himself with nothing and completely debased, he repents, "Father, I have sinned against heaven and against you. I am no longer worthy to be called your son. . . ." He returns home. His father, the perfect image of the heavenly father, embraces him without hesitation. His father is "filled with compassion" and drowns him in gifts. When the older brother becomes angry with jealousy, the father tells him they must "celebrate and be glad, because this brother of yours was dead and is alive again; he was lost and is found."

The message is that no matter what sins we've committed, we can always be transformed, liberated, and purified when we surrender, for we're cleansed by the turning within our own hearts. Like many of us, the prodigal son has to hit bottom before this turning is possible; he has to become desperate before he can surrender. When he does, he is saved. This is the surrender of ishvara pranidhana, total surrender to the Divine.

The message is the same in the *Bhagavad Gita*, too. Krishna tells Arjuna, "Even if you were the most sinful of sinners, Arjuna, you could cross beyond all sin by the raft of spiritual wisdom. . . . Nothing in this world purifies like spiritual wisdom" (4:36).

The Son of the Wind

The rich Indian tradition of storytelling offers us many tales of gods and other celestial beings who descend to Earth and incarnate as earthly creatures like ourselves. Oftentimes, they forget their true Divine nature, believing themselves to be mortals, who like us feel fettered by our limitations and flaws. Having forgotten their Divine nature, they underestimate their own abilities. Sound familiar? They are limited by their own beliefs about themselves—until something happens to wake them up and remind them of who they really are.

Take the beloved little monkey god Hanuman. Hanuman is the son of the wind (*Vayu*), but is born as a *vanara*, or monkey-like person. As a child, Hanuman ran and played in the forest with other vanaras, climbing trees and eating the ripe fruits of the forest. Being the son of the wind, he was fast and powerful, and mischievous! Sometimes he'd grab the forest elephants by their tusks and swing them over his head, or tear up mountains and toss them into the sky. He also liked to taunt the forest-dwelling brahmins. He would douse their sacrificial fires, eat the sacred food left out as offerings to the gods, and pull their beards while they were in their trance-like meditations.

After a while, the brahmins grew fed up with little Hanuman's antics. They pleaded with Lord Brahma, creator of the universe, to curse Hanuman and make him stop bothering them. Lord Brahma could see that Hanuman was causing trouble and was sympathetic to the complaints of the brahmins. But he knew that Hanuman was fundamentally good and destined to be a hero. So Lord Brahma cast a gentle curse. Hanuman would forget his infinite powers and that he was a god. According to the curse, the only way he could remember his powers was when someone else reminded him.

Hanuman went on with his life thinking of himself as just an average little monkey, filled with self-doubts and insecurities, until his life became intertwined with that of Lord Rama, the human incarnation of Vishnu. Vishnu is one of what is sometimes called the Hindu triad or trinity—the three main gods who embody the forces of creation, preservation, and destruction. Brahma creates, Vishnu preserves, and Shiva destroys or transforms. Vishnu has many different *avatars* or incarnations, the most well known probably being Krishna and Rama. It is said that whenever the world is in trouble Vishnu comes to Earth in a different incarnation to help us.

According to Hindu tradition, Lord Rama lived in the second age of man known as the *Treta Yuga*, which followed the *Satya Yuga* of perfect morality. It is said that the Dharma bull, which symbolizes morality, stood on four legs in Satya Yuga, three legs in Treta Yuga, two in the third or *Dvapara Yuga*, and currently, in the immoral age of *Kali Yuga*, on only one.

The story of the life of Lord Rama is the focus of the Hindu epic the *Ramayana*, and Lord Rama is a favorite among Hindus and yogis. Born into a royal family, Lord Rama ultimately ascends to the throne and leads his people into an era of unparalleled harmony and peace. But the reason he's so popular is not simply that he's a good king, but that before he took the throne, he underwent a long period of human suffering. He's popular because we can relate to his struggles, and he gives us hope that we can escape them, too.

Lord Rama's wife Sita (incarnation of the goddess Lakshmi) is kidnapped by a lustful demon named Ravana and taken to a mythical island, which is commonly identified as Sri Lanka. Rama seeks the aid of the monkey army, including Hanuman. In their search for Sita, the vanaras reach the southern tip of India, where they encounter the vastness of the sea, which separates India from Sri Lanka. Seeing the great distance to the other shore, they all grow disheartened by their inability to traverse the water. At that moment of total despair, the other vanaras begin to encourage Hanuman: "You can do it, Hanuman-ji! You're the son of the wind!" And Hanuman begins to remember. As he remembers, his powers (which were never really lost, just forgotten) are restored. He turns himself into a giant and spans the ocean in one great leap, ultimately saving Sita and reuniting her with Lord Rama.

We are all Hanuman. Yoga helps us to remember who we really are: to remember that we're Divine, and to see this same divinity in all living beings.

Milarepa

The life of the Tibetan yogi Milarepa offers us another story of a great sinner who becomes a great saint.[9] Milarepa is a historical figure, though his life story was passed down orally for many centuries before being committed to writing, so it's hard to say which parts of his story are "real" and which are embellishments. As with all teachings, what is real will depend on what resonates as truth, which is not something limited to or fully revealed by the facts. Often, we discover greater truth and wisdom outside of historical facts than we do within them.

Most sources say Milarepa was born in western Tibet in 1052 c.e., although some sources place his birth in 1040. He was born into a large and wealthy family, including an adoring younger sister and two loving parents. The first years of his life were blessed with abundance, good fortune, and great happiness until his father became very ill. Before he died, he entrusted the family's estate to his brother and sister until Milarepa was of age to run it himself. But Milarepa's aunt and uncle were greedy and selfish, and as soon as Milarepa's father died, they began treating Milarepa and his mother and sister with outright disdain and cruelty, forcing them to live in servants' quarters and giving them little food on which to survive.

Finally, when Milarepa came of age, his mother asked her in-laws to honor her dead husband's wishes and turn the estate over to her son. But Milarepa's aunt and uncle refused, throwing them out into the streets, where they were homeless, forced to beg for food, and truly miserable. In her desperation, Milarepa's mother became consumed by anger and hatred and sent Milarepa off to study sorcery, so he could seek revenge on his aunt and uncle. His mother swore she'd kill herself if he didn't avenge them.

Milarepa went in search of a teacher of the black arts, eventually finding a sorcerer who entrusted him with powerful secret teachings and rituals. Using his new powers, Milarepa cast a spell that caused a house to collapse on his entire extended family, killing everyone except for his aunt and uncle, who had to live so they might suffer their loss of family and fortune.

Milarepa's mother was still not satisfied, however. She urged him to cause yet more destruction. Again practicing his black magic, Milarepa conjured hailstorms that destroyed all the village's crops. When he overheard some of the villagers talking about the destruction, he suddenly realized what terrible things he'd done and was filled with remorse.

Milarepa returned to his teacher burning with guilt and regret. The sorcerer realized that Milarepa was being called to a different path, so he sent him to find a teacher of the Dharma. Following his intuitions, Milarepa eventually did: the great Buddhist teacher Marpa the Translator. Marpa accepted him, but subjected him to a series of seemingly endless and cruel trials. Milarepa endured severe hardships at the beginning of his instruction, which proved to Marpa the extent of his commitment and devotion to the path of Dharma.

In order to practice the teachings more deeply, Milarepa ventured alone into the Himalayas, where he lived in a cave for many years, letting go of all worldly attachments, devoting himself completely to the path of liberation, and achieving enlightenment in this lifetime. Milarepa left behind many lyrical poems that remain treasured in Tibetan culture:

> If you lose all differentiation between yourselves and others, fit to
>   serve others you will be.
> And when in serving others you will win success, then shall you
>   meet with me;
> And finding me, you shall attain Buddhahood.[10]

Like so many others, Milarepa's story shows us that no matter what we've done or what's been done to us, we're never so far gone that we can't wake up in this very moment. The yogic teachings tell us that the true Divine Self within remains as pure as a lotus flower growing from the mire. The lotus is naturally found in mucky ponds. From that filth grows this symbol of purity and awakening compassion. As it rises up from the mud, the dirty water beads and falls off its immaculate leaves. The filth can't stick or stain the lotus, though the flower is in the midst of it. The lotus, like us, is always pure.

The Ultimate Cleanse: Love

It's said in Buddhism that all beings contain this lotus of the heart. It begins unopened. As we cultivate the qualities of the Buddha, awaken and open the heart, the lotus unfolds. The opening of the heart lotus represents the awakening of love in our hearts. As we awaken our hearts through love, we find the true purity and true happiness and wholeness we've been seeking.

The Four Immeasurable Minds of Love

Cultivating love for all beings is the key to our own peace of mind. Love is the great antidote to all of our negativity, impurity, and suffering. In his translation and commentary on Patanjali's sutras, Swami Satchidananda stresses that one sutra in particular is of the highest importance in our yogic journeys:

In relationships, the mind becomes purified by cultivating feelings of friendliness towards those who are happy, compassion for those who are suffering, goodwill towards those who are virtuous, and neutrality towards those we perceive as wicked or evil.[11]

These are the Four Immeasurable Minds of Love taught by the Buddha. Swami Satchidananda said that this sutra was for him the "guiding light toward a life of peace and joy." This teaching once again reminds us of our interconnection with all beings. As the Dalai Lama says, "If you want others to be happy practice compassion; and if you want yourself to be happy, practice compassion."[12]

Buddhists describe enlightenment as *bodhicitta*, which translates as an "awakened heart and mind," or a "totally open and aware heart." The Buddhist nun Pema Chödrön refers to bodhicitta as the "soft spot" within our hearts, a place as tender as an open wound.[13] Bodhicitta is the working together of wisdom and compassion. It is the wish to achieve enlightenment, to wake up, in order to help other beings. Those who follow this path are called *bodhisattvas*. The bodhisattva's sole purpose is to help release others from misery. We are surrounded by many bodhisattvas in our world, from aid workers who risk their lives to bring medicine and food to war victims, to nurses and teachers in inner cities, the volunteers walking dogs at the shelters, all those dedicated animal activists who forgo material pleasures in order to alleviate the distress of others, and any one of us who intentionally places ourselves in the midst of suffering in order to bring relief. We all have the capacity to be bodhisattvas.

In the Mahayana school of Buddhism, the practice of the Four Immeasurable Minds of Love is the basis for cultivating bodhicitta and living the life of a bodhisattva.

The Four Immeasurables are:

1. *Maitri* or Loving Kindness: This is the feeling a mother has for her child, or a child might have for an aging parent; a heartfelt desire for that other to be happy and fulfilled.

2. *Karuna* or Compassion: This is deep concern for another's suffering. More than just sympathy, it implies action. If my mother were being tortured, I wouldn't sit on my hands and feel bad for her. I'd get up and help in any way I could. This is karuna. In the *Lotus Sutra*, the bodhisattva Avalokiteshvara (or Avalokita for short, and in China known as Guanyin or Kwan Yin) is described as "looking with the eyes of compassion and listening deeply to the cries of the world." Avalokita is regarded as the epitome of karuna.

3. *Mudita* or Joy: When we practice mudita, we share others' happiness and we wish joy for all. It's the feeling we have when someone for whom we have unconditional love experiences happiness. When our children or our pets run and play and are in great health, we experience a vicarious joy through them: mudita. However, oftentimes, when we see others experiencing happiness, we can become envious or judgmental. Mudita is the antidote to the demon of jealousy.

4. *Upeksha* or Equanimity: This is sometimes misunderstood as a cold indifference to others, but rather it can be understood as the ability to see all beings as equals and equally deserving of love. Equanimity is sometimes described as the fertile soil needed in order to grow good crops. Equanimity is the soil necessary to cultivate the other minds of love. The more balanced and in harmony we are with others, the more relaxed our minds will be. The more distressed and biased we are about others, the more restless the mind. Equanimity helps us release aversion to some beings, as well as attachment. It can be understood as loving detachment for all beings.

Contemplating the fluidity of our relationships and feelings can help us cultivate equanimity. Someone we dislike one day can become a dear friend the next, and someone we feel great affection for one day can be a source of hatred the next.

Virtually every one of the one million divorces that take place in the United States alone every year is a representation of this fluidity.

It also helps to remind ourselves that the greatest teachers are frequently those who push our buttons the most. They help bring out our "issues" and challenge us to work through them. They cause us to see those destructive qualities within ourselves we'd prefer to ignore, but which we cannot release until we see. As we realize that even those for whom we feel aversion help us in some way, we might loosen up a bit as we see the interchangeability of relationships, the impermanence inherent in them all.

Equanimity can also help us deal with our feelings toward difficult people in our lives, even those who harm us or others. In the face of aggression, we can step back enough to try to understand the causes and conditions that gave rise to the aggression or other difficult behavior or quality we're reacting to. We remind ourselves that the real purpose of cultivating bodhicitta is to be of better service to others, to be more peaceful in order that we may be more useful. Letting go of our hatred and anger will benefit all beings, as well as ourselves. Thich Nhat Hanh stresses that if we look deeply enough we can understand that each person is the product of causes and conditions, and with understanding, compassion naturally arises. When we realize that if the aggressors in our world were at peace they would no longer do harm, we'll recognize that if we truly desire a peaceful world, we can only wish for their peace.

My father is skeptical about this stuff. Whenever I talk about extending compassion to all sentient beings, he likes to bring up Hitler and challenge me about whether I think we should have compassion for someone as evil as he. Ultimately, the answer is *yes*. But we start where we are by connecting with the love we already have access to and then growing that love out, little by little, to the extent of our own current capacity. It's the same as if we walked into a gym with no prior weight-lifting experience and tried to lift two hundred pounds. It would be far better to begin with something we could handle and with regular practice we'd develop muscle strength and gradually increase our lifting capacity. The same holds true for our spiritual practices.

In order to benefit from the teaching on the Four Immeasurables we must actually practice them. They aren't something we can simply read about and intellectualize. When we meditate on the Four Immeasurables, we're really setting out with the intention of opening up and finding our tender spots, and lowering the walls we've built up around those places that prevent us from tapping into the sea of peace and love within. We practice learning how to stay with our tenderness and allowing it to transform us into true peace warriors instead of running away and hiding in fear of the pain that's so essential for the transformation of our suffering.

When we work on cultivating the Four Immeasurables, the practice is usually to begin with a beloved. The traditional Buddhist instruction is to start with our mothers, assuming we've had a nurturing, loving mother. If not, we can start with any being for whom we have real, tender, unselfish, unconditional love. Then we move to ourselves, then a friend, and then someone toward whom we have neutral feelings. Then we move to an enemy—or if we're not quite ready for that, someone who pushes our buttons, and we can work up to enemies in time. For example, I'd begin by cultivating a feeling of loving kindness for my mother, and then the wish that she be free from suffering. I'd cultivate a sense of empathetic joy and wish her the peace of equanimity. I would then do the same for each other category, ultimately extending those wishes out to all beings.

The Four Immeasurables are expressed in the following prayer:

> May all sentient beings thrive, may they be happy and healthy;
> May all sentient beings be free of suffering and its causes;
> May all sentient beings know joy;
> May all sentient beings abide in the peace of equanimity, free of
> bias, attachment, and anger.

We want to notice when our hearts shut down because these are the areas where our work lies. And we want to notice what causes our hearts to burst open because we can also use these triggers as tools to help ourselves get unstuck when the heart

Meditation on the Four Immeasurables

- Come to a comfortable seated posture and take a few moments to deepen the breath, relax the body, and still the mind.

- Imagine a river and two banks. On one side is darkness and disease and suffering of all kinds. On the other side is light. Peace and love reign, and there's never any suffering.

- You see all of your loved ones on the dark side of the river crying for help.

- Imagine yourself forming a raft with your own body, expanding so that all your loved ones climb aboard.

- Then imagine that you look to the bank and see your friends and neutral people, and you see them suffering as well. You manage to expand yourself a little more so that they too can fit.

- Then you look back and see the animals on the factory farms, the child soldiers, and the sex slaves. And you continue expanding so they can all climb on and you can ferry them to the other side to this land of Pure Bliss, where they'll never again suffer, and be happy and filled with joy and respect for all other beings.

- Now you can maybe imagine that you look back and see all the beings that cause harm, and you have such clear vision that you can see the causes of their own misery, how they have suffered, too. You can see the conditions that damaged them.

- As you extend your compassion to them, the basic seed of goodness within them grows so that they become again as small children, innocent and filled with love. *(contd.)*

- Now imagine your raft becomes so big it encompasses the whole planet. You take in all humans and animals and all of nature, and you shelter the Earth within you, ferrying all beings to another realm where suffering doesn't exist and all beings treat others with kindness and love.
- Continue in silent meditation for as long as you wish.

does shut down. The Tibetan Buddhist teacher Chögyam Trungpa Rinpoche had an experience when he was young where he witnessed some boys beating and stoning a tiny puppy to death. This apparently had a great effect on him, and he used this experience through his life to open his heart when he felt it had closed down. The Vajrayana school of Buddhism that he taught emphasizes that everything in life can be used like this to help us on our paths.

Two Pillars of Spiritual Practice: Compassion and Peace

There is tremendous pain in this world, and we can deal with this fact in one of three ways. We can shut our eyes and our hearts completely, so we can function; we

Exercise in Cultivating Bodhicitta
What Breaks Our Hearts Open

- Come to a comfortable seated position and take a few moments to relax the body. Find your breath and begin to slow it down. After a few slow, deep breaths, as you begin to relax deepen the breath further by coming to a three-part yogic breath. Begin by inhaling into the abdomen and allowing the belly to swell; deepen the breath by drawing it into the middle and then the upper chest, fully expanding the lungs as you do; exhale by deflating the upper chest, middle chest, and belly. *(contd.)*

- Find the quiet in between the thoughts. Find the vast spaciousness of mind. Breathe into the heart and notice what happens as you encounter the following suggestions:

  - Your mother
  - Your father
  - Your spouse or partner
  - A pet you have now or had as a child
  - A calf taken from his mother
  - The mother of the calf
  - Squirrels playing around the trunk of a tree
  - A terrorist
  - That same terrorist when you learn that before he became a terrorist his family was killed by a bomb dropped by the country he now terrorizes
  - That terrorist when he is sentenced to death for his crimes
  - Losing your first tooth
  - A friend winning the lottery
  - Your worst enemy winning the lottery
  - A primate being experimented on in a laboratory
  - A child falling down and scraping his knee
  - Turtles laying eggs on a beach under the full moon
  - A young orphaned child in a refugee camp
  - A man abusing his wife
  - The abused wife
  - Your beloved running on a beach, in perfect health and filled with peace and joy *(contd.)*

- Yourself running on a beach with your beloved, in perfect health and filled with peace and joy*

- As you follow the suggestions, continue to breathe into the heart. Notice whether the heart expands or contracts, and the temperature and energy you feel. Stay with the sensations, noticing when you want to run or shut down. Do your best to stay and breathe into the sensations without story lines. We want to understand what helps us open our hearts and what causes us to shut down. Sometimes, we shut down in aversion; sometimes, because of too much grief. Maitri counsels us to accept where we are and not force ourselves to take on more than we can handle.

- *   Note what suggestions caused your heart to open, and use these as a can opener for your heart in times when you feel shut down.

can absorb every drop of it personally and succumb to darkness and despair; or we can do everything we need to do to maintain our peace so we're able to keep our hearts open and serve others in need, without shutting down, breaking down, or bringing our own neurosis into the world.

Compassion

Anyone brave enough to face the massive anguish in this world, and who can bear to do that without building a concrete wall around the heart, will at some time feel despair and anger. In this age, where every moment of misery on this planet is instantly and incessantly transmitted, it's easy to become overwhelmed. Most of us aren't strong enough to face the suffering with open eyes, which is why so much continues. The world isn't filled with sadists; it's filled with people who look the other way. Albert Einstein said, "The world is a dangerous place, not because of those who do evil, but because of those who look on and do nothing."[14] This is a call to action. You cannot drown! The world doesn't need us to be anything other than who we are. But we cannot be true to ourselves if we've shut down, broken down, or become consumed by our own darkness. The world needs us to stay awake and keep our hearts open. In order to do that, we must take care of ourselves.

I used to feel that I needed to agonize in solidarity with all those beings tormented so terribly at any given moment, and that taking care of myself was the height of selfishness. I remember thinking that if an animal could endure the torture of a CAFO or fur farm; if a child soldier could withstand the loss and violence that is all he knew; if a woman forced into sexual slavery could bear the shame and abuse that offends all sense of goodness in the world—I couldn't possibly in good conscience allow myself to care for myself or enjoy my life. The least I could do, I felt, was bear witness and suffer with them vicariously.

Thich Nhat Hanh says that our compassion is what connects us with the Buddha within. Our compassion is noble; it links us to other beings. The more we've suffered, the more we can understand the suffering of others. But, he says, "[o]ur suffering is holy if we embrace it and look deeply into it. If we don't, it isn't holy at all. We just drown in the ocean of our suffering."[15]

If we are aware and keep our eyes open, we may watch the evening news on any given night and see things that make us cry in horror and heartbreak. We may scream, rage, and become mad with anger at the injustice and cruelty of the world. The world may appear to us a cold, hostile place, where atrocities aren't just commonplace but woven into the fabric of society. As a result, we could become bitter, despondent, depressed, self-righteous, and unpleasant to be around—injecting our own darkness back into the world.

Alternatively, we might close our eyes, block out the horrors, withdraw inward, and try to ignore them. How do we live in a world with ethnic cleansing, child soldiers, sex slaves, chemical warfare, animal cruelty, and elder abuse? How can this not overwhelm the conscience? "I don't want to know," we say, "I can't handle it."

Yet, when we close our eyes and barricade our tender hearts, we cast darkness over our inner light. This keeps us in an endless cycle of personal suffering—where in order to live with this denial, we must numb ourselves. Some of us turn to drugs, alcohol, overeating, compulsive shopping, or many other externally focused pleasure-seeking behaviors. The result is that we relate to our children, parents, spouses, and friends half-heartedly; the fullness of our hearts is as inaccessible to us as it is to those we love. We are deadened, bored, and dissatisfied. In time, we slide into depression. In our attempt to avoid the pain and suffering of awareness, we become alienated from ourselves and by extension from others as well.

The Buddha exemplifies how it's possible to live in a world full of suffering without becoming depressed, hardened, angry, numb, or self-loathing. He shows us how to live in this world with open eyes and an open heart. Despite—or rather, *because of*—all of the misery in the world, we cannot allow ourselves to be consumed by darkness. We must do whatever it takes to stay connected to our light and bring it into the world. Our nature is light; we need only be true to our nature. Our empathy and compassionate actions can help ease the suffering of others, but our agony cannot. We cannot create a peaceful world through rage and hopelessness. We begin to release ourselves from guilt when we see this, and seeing this, we can begin to treat ourselves with kindness and compassion.

We need to stay connected enough to the world so we know how we can help; so we know the impact our actions and choices have on others; so our hearts remain tender and we can make wise, compassionate decisions. It's important to understand where our food comes from and if living beings were harmed to make it; where our clothing comes from, and whether people or the planet was harmed in its manufacture.

But there's a line between information and masochism. Once we know enough to make informed choices, it's important that we learn to look away. I don't mean burying our heads in the sand, but tormenting ourselves with images and information about suffering doesn't do anyone any good. We need to feel and cry and hurt for the world. But we also need to limit our exposure to what drags us into depression and anger and know when to retreat and heal ourselves. Long before the undertow of despair begins to suck us down, we need to stop and take care of our own needs, or we'll be pulled out to sea before we know it. And we won't do anyone any good then.

Peace

Sri Swami Satchidananda said, "When anything comes to you, first ask yourself, 'Will I be maintaining my peace by getting this, or will my peace be disturbed?' Ask that question for everything—people you will be with, possessions you would like to acquire. Prior to doing anything, ask yourself 'Will this rob me of my peace?' If the answer is yes, then you should choose peace first. Always choose peace. But, if the answer is, 'My peace will not be disturbed by this,' then you can go ahead and still maintain your peace. That should be our aim."[16]

We give energy to what we pay attention to. Therefore, we must make a special effort not to overlook the good that exists in everything and everyone, no matter how small. Even our racist, chauvinistic uncle, who derides us for being gay or vegetarian or Buddhist, has a soft spot. He loves something or someone; he's been hurt somewhere along the way. Maybe he helped a woman exit a violent relationship, or last winter rescued a baby squirrel who fell from his nest. Rather than focusing on the bad we perceive, let's look for the good that's in there somewhere.

I was driving once when I came upon a woman who'd parked in the median and was running up the road with a box in her hand. As I approached, she bent down and gathered up a small bird who was injured. At once, I felt both sorrow for the bird's suffering and gratitude and reverence for the compassion of the woman trying to save him. She gave me hope. I drove away and wept for it all with a smile and a pounding heart. This is life. Coming to terms with life means taking it all in, the "good" and the "bad."

In order to help the world, we must first find our own peace and make it our priority. Every day, we need to go within to a place of peace and quiet. Often, when I meditate in the mornings, as my heart reopens, I end up crying, for my own little sorrows and the suffering of all beings. But after the tears, there's always a golden peace. Although that peace is always there, we forget it as soon as the doorbell rings, or the dog barks, or the baby cries. This is why it's so important to do the things throughout the day, every day, that remind us of that peace within that gives us the strength and joy to get out of bed every morning. I've already highlighted many practices that can reconnect us with our peace. Simply breathing consciously and deeply can be enough. And daily meditation is invaluable as a way of being with ourselves fully.

If we are mindful, we'll learn the wisdom to stay on this side of desperation. We must watch ourselves vigilantly, using the two pillars of compassion and peace to help us navigate life. When the heart closes, it's time to reopen. When the tenderness becomes unbearable, we must turn ourselves again to the light, always remembering the words of Martin Luther King Jr., "Darkness cannot drive out darkness; only light can do that. Hate cannot drive out hate; only love can do that." The world needs our light. It needs our love. So let us be light. Let us be love.

Dissolving the Illusion of Separateness

When we look at the world's terrible injustices and violence, it's natural to want to blame others for the world's ills: "He did it," "They did it," "She did it," "It's his fault, their fault, her fault, God's fault," "I didn't do it," "I'd never do that." The reality— and not some New-Age, hocus-pocus reality, but the objective fact—is that we aren't separate from the world. The hatred and bigotry that cause wars and oppression on the other side of the globe begin with anger, hostility, resentment, or greed within ourselves. The Buddha taught that we have the seeds of all mental formations and emotions within us. Those seeds that we water will flourish; those we starve will lie dormant; but they're all there. We cannot understand each other until we understand ourselves deeply; we cannot have compassion for others until we find it for ourselves.

The world isn't separate from us. We know this, because no matter how hard we try to shut it out it gets in one way or another. When we watch the evening news, our hearts either burst with sympathy and tenderness, or shut down and harden to what we see happening "out there" to "them." Either way, we're affected. How we react is our choice, but we can't simply block out the world: it's already within us. Sages and mystics have told us for millennia that the world without is within. As the Sufi poet Rumi mused, "You are the mighty ocean in the drop."[17]

Yoga teaches us that the greatest obstacle to union and peace is the illusory idea of separateness, which causes our alienation from one another. We see ourselves as separate and different. We compete with, compare ourselves to, and judge one another. World peace begins when we look within with honesty and embrace what we find with understanding and loving kindness.

We must be gentle with ourselves to be gentle with the world. If we're hard on ourselves, we'll be hard on others. Only when we really understand ourselves can we understand others. This means being honest: our warts, pimples, and all. Rather than pretending they're not there because we're ashamed, we need to embrace them with awareness and understanding—to look deeply into our own pettiness, jealousy, impatience, anger, greed, desire, or whatever our particular neuroses are until we can discern the need that causes them. Every neurosis stems from some need, emptiness, loneliness, or fear.

Once we allow ourselves to feel this underlying longing, we can understand ourselves better and treat ourselves more gently and compassionately. Only then can we begin to understand and find real compassion for those "others," with all their warts. Rather than looking at the world and seeing how divided we are and how awful *they* are, we can look within and engage those parts of ourselves we've been hiding and bring them into the light of awareness, under which they are stripped naked and purified. To find true, lasting peace within ourselves and in the world, we must work with reality.

Gandhi is reported to have said we must "be the change we want to see in the world." This implies first that we look within, transform the resentments of the past and fears for the future, and lower whatever barriers we've built around our own hearts. Only then can we turn to the world we live in and really *see* the other living beings with whom we share this reality—treating them with respect and practicing compassion in our actions.

Tonglen

A Buddhist meditation practice called *Tonglen*, or taking and sending, can help us dissolve these barriers. The eighth-century Buddhist monk Shantideva, author of *The Way of the Bodhisattva*, a comprehensive manual for leading the life of the bodhisattva, tells us that:

> He who desires shelter quickly
> For himself and for all others
> Should use this sacred mystery
> The exchanging of himself for others.[18]

In Tonglen, we learn to dissolve our boundaries with others by going directly against our habitual, selfish instincts to reject the negativity of others and guard our own good. Tonglen is often folded into a formal meditation practice, but some traditions incorporate it into every breath. The idea is that as we inhale, we take in whatever is disturbing another, and as we exhale, we send out the specific relief he or she needs. In this way, we incorporate in each breath of our lives our deep aspiration to serve other beings and to liberate them from suffering.

The instructions are usually to begin with some being we already have great tenderness for, just like when we practice the Four Immeasurables. If my grandfather has painful arthritis, I might inhale all his pain and exhale relief. From a place of tangible tenderness, we begin to extend ourselves further. If the neighbor starts pounding on our front door, shouting about our tree falling on his fence, we might inhale his rage and exhale peace. We take on experiences and transform them within ourselves. We're able to do this because we have a limitless source of love and peace within, enough to transform any experience.

In this way, we can use any situation, including our own emotions, to connect with other beings at any given moment. If I've been cheated on and dumped for another woman and my heart is broken, I can call to mind all the other lonely people in the world, inhaling all of our loneliness together and sending out the relief they need as I exhale. In so doing, I link my suffering with that of many others. As I do, I realize I'm not alone. And as I transform their pain and send out the fullness and love they need, I also am filled. We can connect with all other beings in the same way no matter what the situation, including in moments of joy. If I'm sitting at the dinner table eating a vegan feast with my loving family, I can pause and wish that all beings were free from hunger and that they, too, might know security, freedom, and love.

This very gentle, loving practice helps us accept ourselves and others. We can use every experience as an opportunity for dissolving the barriers that separate us from others.

Establishing a Meditation Practice

"Give us this day our daily bread. . . ." For many years, when I heard the Lord's Prayer, I thought of this line as an antiquated remnant of an anachronistic church with which I felt no real connection. Then I heard a very wise minister explain that just

Meditation: Emptiness and Tonglen (Taking and Sending)

Find a comfortable seated posture. Relax the body. Begin to deepen the breath.

Emptiness
- Watch the breath and notice the gaps between the thoughts. Focus on these gaps. Try to keep the mind focused on the breath for ten breaths. *(contd)*.

- Notice every time the mind wanders, and gently, nonjudgmentally, bring the awareness back to the breath, to the space.
- Allow the space between the thoughts to expand. Breathe into a vast, limitless space.
- When words arise, allow them to dissolve as quickly as they came, returning over and over to the breath. Practice breathing into this spacious, peaceful void for a few minutes, allowing all concepts, ideas, and words to evaporate continually into the ether—even allowing your sense of your own body to blur until it, too, evaporates.

Taking and Sending
- Call to mind someone very dear to you who's experiencing any difficulty or suffering. As you inhale, take in all of his or her pain and suffering. As you draw in that pain and suffering, imagine it as thick black smoke. Feel what that feels like.
- Allow that energy to be transformed by your limitless love for this other being. As you exhale, release pure peace and love, all the goodness you have inside of you, giving that to your beloved.
- With each inhalation, draw in his or her pain. Imagine you're swallowing the poison so the other person doesn't have to. Your love and the boundless light within you are so powerful that the black smoke and suffering are transformed. With each exhalation, you release pure golden rays of soothing, peaceful light.
- Alternate between resting your awareness in the pure, spacious void with periods of taking and sending.
- Finish the practice with resting in the void.

like the bread we eat, our spiritual practices become stale and we need to replenish them on a daily basis. Meditation today, no matter how transcendent, isn't going to carry us over. We need a daily practice if we are to stay spiritually fresh.

Our whole society is built on an obsession with distracting ourselves from our selves. We fear quiet, solitude, emptiness. The trick is that emptiness isn't really empty! When we empty ourselves of all of our ideas and conceptions, we empty ourselves of limitations. When we let go of our perceptions of the world, we let go of the walls and barriers and the smallness of ego, and open to the vast fullness of the Divine within and without: everywhere.

We must become able to sit still with ourselves, to be present with the feelings that roll through and wash over us, as we sit still and breathe and allow them to pass, without clinging to or chasing it. If we can do this, the waves will pass as surely as they do in the ocean. When we deny or suppress or run from those waves of feeling, they build until they are a tidal tsunami in which we drown.

When we allow ourselves to be present to the feelings and breathe through them, they soften and begin to dissolve. We see they aren't fixed or permanent. Nothing is. So, too, when we're riding high on a wave; we know that wave will crash—with a gentle rolling fall or with great force. The crash is a lot less startling if we can stay connected to something in the center of the wave that neither ascends nor descends. When we crash, as we will, we can fall in the comforting knowledge that the defeat, however crushing, will also pass and wash over us as we prepare to catch the next wave.

Up and down. This is life. The model yogi sits in the center, perfectly in equilibrium as the pendulum of external circumstances swings wildly from one side to the other. We can achieve this if we choose. But there are other models, too. Some prefer the center; others ride the highs and lows but with knowledge of the center, experiencing the turbulence with enough detachment to remain connected to the core of peace.

All of the spiritual traditions emphasize the importance of staying in the present. So many of our fears are about the past or future. But the formal practices are where we recharge to interact with the world from a place of peace, understanding, tolerance, and compassion. We can take what we practice and bring it into the world in all of our thoughts, words, and actions. This is the true meaning of mindfulness. The world is our greatest teacher, as well as our greatest test. Throughout the day, we can pay attention and notice when we feel we're drifting from the center of peace. When we observe fear rising up, we can see where the mind has gone and draw ourselves back to the now.

If we're just beginning a meditation practice, it's best to start simply, even for two minutes at the beginning. As we become more comfortable with the practice, we can increase to five-minute periods, then ten, fifteen, twenty, up to half an hour in a sitting. Early morning is an ideal time to meditate, before the sun rises, when the world and the mind are calm. The mind is also naturally calm near sunset, making dusk another ideal time for meditation. However, if these times don't work for you, you can meditate at any hour. Nonetheless, it's helpful to establish a routine, meditating in the same place and the same time every day.

Our meditation space can be as simple as a corner in our bedroom, but we'll want it to be out of the way of commotion of family, friends, pets, or society. We could meditate in the middle of a city sidewalk, but that's probably not ideal. The ancient sages tell us to find a quiet space free from distractions. And we want to be comfortable. If you are healthy without any major health problems, try sitting cross-legged on the floor with a small blanket or pillow under your hips. If that is a strain for you, you can use a meditation bench or a regular chair.

I like to use a timer when I meditate, so my mind can focus on something other than how long I've been sitting. It's helpful to have a designated space devoted to your practices. This might be an altar where you can place any images that help you center and focus your practice. You might have images of Jesus, if that is whom you identify with; Guanyin, the bodhisattva of compassion; St. Francis of Assisi; the Buddha; or a pet cat you had as a child. Any symbols that help you focus your mind on opening your heart and reconnecting with the Divine Self will do.

It's natural to be apprehensive, but in time this dissolves, as meditation becomes a habit. Then, even if you still feel reluctant, you do it anyway. Eventually, you'll come to your meditation cushion with enthusiasm, knowing how much sweetness exists on the other side of whatever we're afraid to sit with, and that sitting through it is the only way to get to the sweetness. Most people have some idea about what meditation is supposed to be, or they have no idea but still think there is such knowledge out there in the universe. There is no one-size-fits-all meditation technique or right way to meditate. There are many different styles and techniques, and you may need to experiment to find what works for you.

Meditation usually begins with cultivating one-pointed concentration on one object of meditation. That object can be the breath, a *mantra* like the sacred syllable *Om*, or a particular deity, the light within, a candle, or an image eliciting memory of the character of the Divine Self. Over time, the object may drop away so only pure consciousness remains. Don't be discouraged if this doesn't happen immediately. In some traditions we might begin by focusing on emptiness, space, the great limitless void. Sometimes, we use techniques designed to awaken certain feelings or states of mind, such as compassion or loving kindness for all beings. Ramana Maharshi, one of the great modern enlightened masters, recommended self-inquiry in meditation, a constant probing with the question "Who Am I?" He taught that this question would ultimately lead us to see the nonexistence of the "I" and to realize the Divine Self, thereby leading us to the attainment of liberation.

The Basic Meditation Technique

- Find a quiet place; sit upright, but comfortably. Perhaps slide a pillow or blanket under your hips to elevate them just above the knees.
- Close your eyes and begin to notice how the body feels. Notice where you're holding tension through the body: scan the hips, belly, shoulders,

jaw, face, the temples in particular, and focus on releasing and softening in those areas.

- Find the breath and notice the quality of the breath, then begin to deepen it. Draw the breath up into the belly, fill it, then draw it up into the middle chest and finally the upper chest, fully expanding the lungs. Reverse that process by deflating the upper and then the middle chest and then the belly, drawing the navel back to the spine as you completely exhale. Continue at your own pace, trying to keep the breath as full and deep and slow and steady as is comfortable.

- Notice if thoughts cling in the mind. Become aware of them and then try to step back and watch the thought, creating distance between yourself and it, and then try to let it go.

- Draw the breath up into the heart and feel the sensations. Allow yourself to feel what's there, even if it means becoming emotional. Then come back to the breath and exhale.

- Neither suppress emotions nor attach to them. They come and we allow them to go.

- Breathe in and out of the heart, trying to stay connected to that softness—beyond ego, beyond thought. Find that sweet spot in the center of the heart and let that sweetness fill you. Find fullness and wholeness in that unconditional love, knowing that is the true Self that connects us with all living beings.

- Whenever the mind wanders, try to gently draw yourself back to the breath, to the quiet spaces between the thoughts. Keep relaxing any part of the body, mind, or heart that tenses back up. Keep returning to the breath, to the eternal peace at your core that is always there at the center of the ups and downs.

Whatever way you meditate, the common goal is to quiet and control the discursive mind and bring it into concentration to escape illusion and discover truth. All the contemplative traditions agree that in order to find truth, we must quiet the mind. In the quiet, truth speaks to us without words.

Mantra

A mantra is a sacred word, phrase, or even syllable that evokes the Divine. The repetition of mantra is a practice that brings focus and concentration to the mind and helps us tune into that Divine frequency that's always broadcasting underneath the chatter of our restless minds. It's the bridge that helps us traverse the mind and realign with the Divine within, a form of prayer in the sense that all of our deepest intentions are prayers to the Divine wisdom within our own hearts. The mantra can be recited silently in the mind or recited or sung out loud. When practiced with others, it can be a heart opening and even ecstatic practice of sharing in Divine love. Mantra practice is a simple but powerful tool we can incorporate into our daily lives to purify the mind and cultivate the deep intentions that ultimately drive and shape our lives.

The ancient yogis perceived the universe as being in a state of constant vibration. They understood, as modern science affirms, that sound is how we perceive vibration. Through sound, they teach us, we can bring ourselves into harmony with certain vibrations, and align ourselves with the vibrations of the universe. In this way, we can align our consciousness with the language of the universe.

While there is no adequate direct translation of the word *mantra*,[19] the word itself is derived from the Sanskrit root *man*, which means "to think" and is related to the word *manas*, or "mind," and *tra*, which translates as "instrumentality" or sometimes "protection." Buddhists often use the word in this way, interpreting *mantra* as "mind protecting." Primarily, the mantra protects the mind from itself. Yoga and Buddhism both teach us that the bulk of our suffering comes from our own minds, thoughts, or perceptions (or more often misperceptions). We ruminate and stew and obsess over the wrongs done to us: the missed opportunities, jealousies, anxieties over the future; what we should have said, what bills are overdue, that the dog is sick, or our children are failing out of school. The list goes on *ad infinitum*. When we chant, all of this stops. We focus on the mantra, and in the relative quiet of the mind we transcend all of those tormenting thoughts. It's not that we suppress them; they just naturally dissipate. As we repeat the mantra over and over, the mind holds on to it, aligns itself with it, and brings us closer to its truth. As the Buddha taught, "Our life is shaped by our mind. We become what we think."[20]

We might use mantra as part of a formal practice like we do meditation, setting aside a certain amount of time in the morning or evening to repeat it. But mantra can also be used throughout our days and nights—whenever the mind begins to wander from the present moment and gets us into trouble.

For example, when I'm cooking I often notice my mind drifting off to whatever its latest obsession is. I watch myself becoming upset over something someone said or I didn't say, or something someone else has or I don't have, and I wrestle with my mind to stop having these thoughts. I lose the match over and over. As I prepare the food I'm making, I sense that I'm putting these destructive thoughts and turbulent emotions into the food I'm preparing. (This is why in Ayurvedic cooking it's considered important only to eat food prepared by someone who loves us.) In order to get out of my own head and make sure I'm not feeding emotional poison to my friends and family, I now have a prophylactic practice of mantra-chanting whenever I cook, beginning mantra even before the negative thought-waves arise.

We can use mantra in this way in any situation where we find ourselves becoming consumed with negative, destructive, or unproductive thoughts. Mantra can help us transform the mundane into the sacred, or more precisely to recognize the sacred in what appears mundane when we're not fully present. Mantra is an invaluable tool to help us re-center ourselves in that inner space from which all life can be touched deeply and related to from the heart. Mantra was an essential practice for Gandhi, who explained that in his personal experience, "[t]he mantram becomes one's staff of life and carries one through every ordeal. . . . Each repetition . . . has a new meaning, each repetition carrying you nearer and nearer to God."[21]

Chanting mantras out loud and in a group setting is one of the main practices of *Bhakti Yoga*, or the yoga of devotion. The word *bhakti* derives from the Sanskrit root *bhaj* ("to share" or "to participate in"). Specifically, it refers to the sharing of our own Divine hearts with others. From the perspective of bhakti, association with other spiritual seekers is essential to achieving union with the Divine. One of the main practices of bhakti is *kirtan*. Kirtan involves a call-and-response style of singing mantras and is often accompanied by musical instruments like the harmonium, hand symbols, and drums.

Just like in silent mantra repetition, when we chant out loud, we still the mind and allow ourselves to become absorbed in the Divine presence within our own hearts. Kirtan has the added element of being a shared experience, from which we derive more strength and support in our practice. When we come together to sing the Divine names, we can experience a tremendous sense of connection with others as we share ourselves with a group of people collectively surrendering to the love in our own hearts, a love that removes the barriers that separate us. Bhakti helps us discover the Divine presence within and celebrate that same presence in the hearts of all beings.

Unlike the silent repetition of mantra, vocalizing mantra in a group setting, whether in a kirtan or in a yoga class, is an extroverting practice. It allows us to connect with a community of others. But anytime we open and share our hearts with others we make ourselves vulnerable. I suspect this is why most students coming to a class for the first time are uncomfortable with chanting.

The first time I found myself in a class where I was asked to chant, I had a complete breakdown. I was just beginning my own exploration of the practices of yoga, when I still had a lot of mud to confront before I'd find my lotus, and I some-what blindly signed up for a workshop that combined yoga and dance with mantra. We were asked to do certain postures and then move freely around the room in whatever way we felt drawn to. Later, we sat in a circle and chanted *Om* in the same freestyle way. I remember the people surrounding me seemed to have melodious voices. The sounds coming from their mouths appeared to originate deep in their cores, and they created rich, warm tones.

I, on the other hand, could barely squeeze out a squeak. My voice was trapped in my throat and disconnected from the rest of me. I heard this feeble cry coming out of me and it broke my heart. It was a horrible little whimper like that of a sick child or injured cat. At the time, I was still working as a big firm lawyer. I wasn't afraid to speak my mind and I took great pleasure in winning every argument in my professional and personal life. Yet here I was in this class suddenly strangled by my own insecurity and weakness. I knew how to speak my mind, but apparently not my heart. So I just sat in silent tears as everyone around me continued with their resonant symphony. At the first break, I ran into the bathroom and wept. The rest of the day is a blur, and still a painful memory when I remember how broken I felt at that time.

So I understand when students come into class and sit with furrowed brows, their lips immobile and bodies tense, while the regulars chant with comfortable smiles and sometimes tender tears. I know that what the newcomers don't yet understand is that it doesn't matter what our voices sound like or that we don't really know the words. What matters is that we chant from the heart. Listening to someone chant with a classically beautiful voice can be a stirring and uplifting experience, but the quality of mantra is measured by sincerity and tenderness, surrender and devotion, not our ability to sing at the right pitch or memorize the Sanskrit.

My voice will never be Grammy worthy, but now I can sit at the front of my classes and lead kirtan, singing from the tenderness in my own heart and the bottomless well of love for all beings that soothes, envelops me, and pours out. It doesn't matter what I sound like. Even when my voice cracks or I hear myself hit a "wrong" note, I no longer think I sound awful. I can smile to myself with compassion and the knowledge that real beauty comes from a heart filled with love. As a bonus, the more we chant and the more our hearts open, that freedom releases the tightness in the throat so our voices open up and mature into well-tuned instruments.

For many, hearing Sanskrit chanting reminds us of our own religious backgrounds. For those of us who've had unpleasant experiences in the tradition in which we were raised, the similarity can stir up some unpleasant memories. For some, it's not the similarities but the differences in the practice that cause the discomfort. We may worry that it's sacrilegious to chant to the deities of another religion, that we're worshipping false gods. But remember: from a yogic perspective, the Divine is within. We practice in order to discover that divinity within. When we sing the Divine names, we aren't so much worshipping an external entity as summoning an energy that exists within ourselves as well as throughout the cosmos.

In Indian philosophy, the Divine is seen to exist in all things, to encompass everything. This impersonal divinity is too big for the mind to grasp all at once. So we relate to and embrace different facets of the Divine. We evoke the Divine maternal qualities when we chant to one of the goddesses, or we connect with our ability to overcome and transform obstacles when we chant to Ganesha, the elephant-headed god known for his ability to remove all obstacles. Each deity represents a different aspect of the Divine—one we can grasp, a quality that exists within us and in the world that surrounds us.

Mantras come from all the world's different traditions, so if we connect with a particular tradition, we can adopt a mantra associated with it. We don't have to chant in Sanskrit and we don't have to be Hindu to chant in Sanskrit if we choose to. We can use any word or phrase that helps us connect with the Divine, or God, or Love, or whatever word we choose to attach to the experience of the sacred that transcends us and transforms us, purifies us and makes us whole again, and brings us to a state of equilibrium and harmony within and in relation with everything. Because mantra is a Sanskrit word, outside of the Indian traditions we don't necessarily use the word *mantra*. But the use of a centering word or phrase to help us quiet the mind and connect with the Divine is not unique to the Eastern traditions.

The tradition of mantra in the Christian church goes back many centuries. In the anonymous fourteenth-century mystical work *The Cloud of Unknowing*, the author advises the reader to "[t]ake just a little word, of one syllable rather than of two; for the shorter it is the better it is in agreement with this exercise of the spirit. Such a one is the word 'God' or the word 'love.' Choose which one you prefer, or any other according to your liking—the word of one syllable that you like best. Fasten this word to your heart, so that whatever happens it will never go away. This word is to be your shield and your spear, whether you are riding in peace or in war. With this word you are to beat upon this cloud and this darkness above you. With this word you are to strike down every kind of thought under the cloud of forgetting."[22]

If we have a personal connection with Jesus Christ, we might use the name *Jesus* as our mantra, repeating the holy name silently and holding it in our hearts. Another ancient Christian mantra is the *Maranatha*, an Aramaic phrase translated either as "Come, Lord!" or "Our Lord has come." Probably the most well-known mantra is the syllable *Om*, which though simple is said to contain all other mantras within it, as it represents the sound of the universe—the sound that *is* the universe. The Christian Bible tells us, "In the beginning was the Word, and the Word was with God, and the Word was God" (John 1:1). That word, according to Indian tradition, is *Om*.

Mantra has been used for millennia in many Buddhist traditions as well. Maybe the most common of these is *Om mane padme hum*. It's hard to capture the essence of this (or any) mantra in a literal translation, though the translation of "You are the jewel in the lotus" is quite beautiful. It is said that reciting this mantra invokes the blessings of Chenrezig, otherwise known Avalokiteśvara, or Guanyin, the embodiment of compassion. This mantra is said to encapsulate all of the Buddha's teachings.

More than the literal translation, or even the stories associated with the mantra, the mantra must be understood by a part of our consciousness that exists beyond the constraints of intellect. It must be known intimately, by the heart. This distinction is easier to see in the French language, where there are two separate verbs that translate into the English "to know." *Savoir* means "to know" with the mind, as in knowing a fact; *connaître* means "to know" more as in knowing a person. We might say we come to know mantra more in the sense of *connaître* than *savoir*. And we come to know the meaning of a mantra more in the way we come to know a dear friend, or we come to know the Divine.

Another beautiful Tibetan mantra that captures the ideals of the bodhisattva is *Lokah samastha sukinoh bhavantu.* You can find many different translations, but they all express the basic wish that all beings everywhere be free from suffering; that they live in joy and happiness; that the forces of light in the world overcome the forces of darkness; and that our own thoughts, words, and actions contribute to the liberation of all beings.

In the guru-based spiritual traditions, the guru usually gives the student a personal mantra. But if we don't have a guru, we can also choose our own, allowing the inner guru to choose for us by paying attention to what speaks deeply to us. We can choose a word or phrase that resonates with us and elevates us so we feel ourselves coming into alignment with the higher Self, the sacred and Divine. We can chant whatever it is that touches that mysterious center of our being and brings us to a state of love, or that ineffable peace "that passes all understanding" (Philippians 4:7).

We don't even have to know what the word means, at least not consciously. Often, we find that we deeply understand the meaning of a mantra before we ever learn the translation. The mantra speaks to us at a level beyond the intellect. It pierces the mind and soothes it. As we focus on the mantra the mind is stilled.

Maybe we choose a mantra that represents the name of a god or goddess whose qualities we seek to emulate or bring ourselves into alignment with, or whose blessings we long to receive. Devotees of Lord Krishna believe that chanting the holy names of Krishna is a way for all people to achieve union with the Supreme person, or God. Krishna *is* actually embodied in his name. When we chant Krishna, we associate directly with him. As we chant, we feel him. We experience him. So when we chant the Hare Krishna, the *maha* (great) mantra, we come into union with Krishna himself. We come into union with God:

Hare Krishna Hare Krishna Krishna Krishna Hare Hare
Hare Rama Hare Rama Rama Rama Hare Hare

A powerful and transformative use of the mantra is to repeat it silently to ourselves. This can be done in times of distress, or when we recognize that our thoughts are carrying us to habitual places we'd rather not go, or when we're simply bored and feeling disconnected from the beauty and joy of life. Repeating the mantra is an effective and direct method for reminding ourselves of the Divine presence within, of our connection with the Divine, and even more to the point, of the truth of our own divinity.

We might try chanting many different mantras until one stands out that aligns us with the Divine we recognize within our own souls. Or we may continue to use many mantras that speak to different needs at different times. Many teachers will advise choosing one mantra and sticking with it. Whether we choose one or use several, mantra is most beneficial when we repeat it regularly as part of a daily practice, so it becomes ingrained and we maintain a connection with the Divine at all times. Just like the great spiritual songs sung by African Americans during periods of oppression and slavery, the real power of mantra is its ability to lift us up and connect us with the Divine, to help us transcend our immediate circumstances and link us with great strength, wisdom, and love.

I once heard an interview with a "freedom rider" from the 1960s. She was one of the hundreds of college kids from the North who decided to join the struggle for equality in the South. Civil rights groups visited college campuses and trained the students in nonviolent resistance. She explained that the training basically consisted of volunteers lying on the ground and wrapping their arms around themselves while they were mock-beaten by "police officers." She talked about how intense the training itself was. But it wasn't until they were in the South and fellow freedom riders started getting shot that they realized how serious the reality actually was. She said she felt it was too late to get out at that point, but they were all terribly frightened. They missed their families and worried they'd never see them again. So they sang. They sang the Gospel spirituals, those songs that connected them with a force greater than themselves, and in those songs, sung together, they found peace and the Divine love that gave them the strength to carry on. This is the power of mantra.

Karma Yoga—Selfless Service

> The only ones among you who will be really happy are those who have
> sought and found how to serve.—**Albert Schweitzer**[23]

Being alive means taking action. We all have to act in one way or another. The word *karma* simply means "action." As we know, *yoga* means "union"; therefore, *karma yoga* is the path to union through action, specifically selfless action, or service. Karma yoga is the practice of using our actions as a form of yoga in a way that recognizes and honors the unity and interconnection of all life. According to yogic philosophy, the most perfect action is one that harms no one and ideally helps at least one being.

When we stop seeking our own happiness and begin serving others, our own personal suffering is transformed and our lives take on real meaning. We escape our feelings of smallness. We let go of the pettiness, fear, and resentments that have kept us stuck and held us back from our own limitless potential. In serving and respecting others, we find dignity, courage, and self-love. The most fundamental truth we learn in yoga is that of our connection with all life and all other beings. If we can understand this truth, we can understand all the other teachings. Yoga tells us that if we want to be happy, we must live in harmony with the truth of interconnection.

In the *Bhagavad Gita*, the warrior Arjuna struggles to understand in practical terms how he should actually live in the world if he is ever to obtain peace. He wants to know what he should do, how he should act, and how a righteous person should live. The answer is simple: live for the well-being of others; dedicate your actions to serving others. Krishna says that those who act out of fear, anger, and selfish desires are "utterly deluded, and are the cause of their own suffering." He tells Arjuna that the true path to peace is through karma yoga: "Strive constantly to serve the welfare of the world. . . . Do your work with the welfare of others always in mind. . . . Perform all work carefully, guided by compassion."[24]

Roshan, one of my teachers in India, used to say that once we realize we're all connected, we realize that serving others is serving ourselves. So, he said with a smile, go ahead and be selfish, by serving others.

Think about what it feels like when we're consumed by petty, ego-based desires in that never-ending pursuit of personal gain: whether it's the desire to make more money, to be with a certain person, to get something we want, like a bigger house or a prestigious job. We all know that craving to satisfy some burning and ultimately unquenchable desire. One way to think about these desires is in terms of energy.

In an earlier chapter we touched on the energy vortices through the body that Indian philosophy calls chakras. Each is located near a physical region of the body, though they don't really correspond to anything physical. They are just different psychic energy centers. When we're stuck in the first (the root) chakra, located near the base of the spine, we are locked in fight-or-flight sorts of impulses. Everything becomes about *me* and *mine*, about survival: me or you. *We're on a sinking ship and there's one life preserver, and I'm taking it.* Just thinking about this scenario makes my jaw clench, stomach tighten, and heart shrivel.

When our basic needs are cared for—for instance, when we have food and a house—we're freed up a bit and can start thinking about our next basic biological need: sex and procreation, which are connected with the second chakra. When we're living from our second chakra, we look to gratify our sexual desires, to consume and feed our lust and longing. This can breed all kinds of jealousy and competition and is a continuation of our drive to acquire for our own fulfillment. Our next basic instinct is that of seeking power and control, which are the qualities associated with the third chakra, located near the solar plexus region of the body. From this place, we want money, material possessions, power over others, and control over situations.

All of the first three chakras are very ego-oriented. When we're fixed in any of these three centers, the world appears to be a place with scarce resources, where we seek to get as much for ourselves as we can. It's only when we move to the fourth chakra, located in the heart, that a fundamental shift happens. We begin to release ego-based longing and open into karuna, or compassion, letting go of selfishness so we can give to and serve others in need who suffer. From here, the energy can continue to rise into the higher centers, freeing us to seek out more enlightened pursuits.

As long as we're stuck in the energy of the first three chakras, we remain mired in a scarcity mentality: *I feel impoverished, so I want to take.* When we work only for the fruits of our actions, for a personal reward—whether monetary or in gratitude and compliments—we're never satisfied. We always need more and are trapped in a mindset of limitation and lack. We feel small and petty, and the illusion of separation and alienation from the true, Divine Self is reinforced. We think that if only someone would give us what we want (money, love, fame, attention, etc.) we'd feel whole and elevated, uplifted, happy, and full.

All of the great spiritual teachings tell us that the reverse is true. The more we release ego and small selfish desires, the closer we come to realizing the inherent fullness and endless wealth of the Divine Self within. The sages who wrote the *Upanishads* tell us we *are* our deepest longing. The Buddha taught the same thing. As Thich Nhat Hanh says, "Nirvana teaches us that we already are what we want to become."[25] As we've seen, when we practice the Four Immeasurables we touch this limitless generosity within—this boundless, inexhaustible source of love and everything we truly desire. It is in this spirit that we realize that, to quote St. Francis's famous prayer, "it is in giving that we receive." As we tap into that sense of generosity, we are filled with it. The more we seek to take from others, the more impoverished we feel; the more we give, the richer and fuller we are; the more we seek love, the lonelier we are; the more we give love, the more we're filled with love and the more we realize we *are* love.

Any act without self-interest or seeking anything in return can be considered karma yoga. In Sanskrit, such actions are *nish kama karma*, "action without selfish desire." When we serve others from this true spirit of generosity, we step out of the ego-based fears of poverty and loneliness, of "What about me?" and "Where's my reward?" When we give in the spirit of love and devotion, we reconnect with the true fullness of the Divine Self. We reconnect with the truth of the Self that is always whole and full, pure and light.

Acting selflessly and without desire can sound like deprivation, or a life without passion or interest. The idea of renunciation conjures images of emaciated, wandering ascetics, homeless and without a family; people who've retreated into a cave or a monastery, devoid of any enjoyment of life. Krishna says that the wise person understands that the path of action and the path of renunciation are one and the same. This is true because renunciation is a mental state. It doesn't mean we can't enjoy life or we have to give up family, home, or employment. Yoga is an internal practice. Monks shave their heads and trade in their street clothes for saffron robes as a sign of nonattachment to the ways of the world and their commitment to the spiritual path. But we can just as easily become attached to these symbols if the mind isn't free. Similarly, many people identify themselves with their expensive hairdos, designer boots, or blue jeans. What matters is not what we look like on the outside; it's what's in our mind and our heart that counts.

The true renunciate, the true karma yogi, is always serving, active in the world but free of attachment to the fruits of those actions. Krishna tells Arjuna, "Fill your mind with me, focus every thought on me, think of me always . . . [then] you will be united with me."[26] Does this really mean that we must think of Krishna all the time? Some followers of Krishna certainly believe this, but for the mystic, for the yogi, Krishna represents the Divine in all life. And what is the Divine? It is love. It is the recognition of our connection. It is the dissolution of our ideas of separation. So to keep Krishna in mind at all times is to look deeply into all things in order to see their true and ultimate nature, in order to live in a way that honors each being and all life as an intimate part of ourselves.

Just as the apostle Paul asked the Thessalonians to pray continually, so we can go through our daily lives engaged in normal activities with a constant prayer in the heart and a constant yearning for the Divine, with unbroken reverence and love for all life. Imagine how beautiful our lives could be if we did this: if we looked at all life with the eyes of love and wonder, and a tenderness of heart that kept us open to all. Imagine being completely present in each moment—fully awake, plugged in, and engaged with every leaf blowing in the wind, every dragonfly buzzing by, every precious moment with our loved ones, every miraculous breath of life.

Instead of selfless service and renunciation as gray and drab, passionless or without enjoyment, the yogis mean letting go only of the selfish desires that keep us imprisoned in a constrained understanding of reality where we feel disconnected and unfulfilled. When we live to serve, our desire to know our own Divine nature burns stronger than ever. Our wish to see and merge with the Divine and to serve the Divine in other beings stirs us to life. Our love for others and the planet, our appreciation of the beauty and impermanence of life, our sense of how we use our limited time caring for those who need our help: these desires continue to grow and evolve within us, driving us to immerse ourselves in our love for this world. In his introduction to the *Bhagavad Gita*, Eknath Easwaran explains that "the man or woman who realizes God has yoked all human passions to the overriding desire to give and love and serve; and in that unification we can see, not the extinction of personality, but its full blossoming. This is what it means to be fully human. . . ."[27]

If we still feel dubious that selflessness is truly the path to happiness, we can turn to modern science for reassurance. In a multitude of studies, researchers have found that volunteering provides significant and tangible benefits not just to those served, but to those doing the service. Studies show a wide range of benefits experienced by people who volunteer regularly, including lower cholesterol, greater happiness, less pain, lower blood pressure, and even longer lives.[28]

Further studies on the impact of love, compassion, generosity, and kindness show that these altruistic emotions reduce stress in the body and increase immunity.[29] Even just thinking kind thoughts can have physiological benefits. Subjects in one study were shown a film of Mother Teresa working with the poor in Calcutta. Those who merely watched the film demonstrated significant increases in protective antibodies associated with improved immunity. Subjects who were shown other films showed no such antibodies. The researchers thus concluded that simply "dwelling on love strengthened the immune system."[30]

The theory of karma tells us that all of our actions have an effect, a reaction, like a boomerang. When we do something good it comes back to us; when we do something harmful, that too comes back to us one way or another. Modern science agrees. When we help others, we ourselves benefit in mind and body. This idea is well understood by members of twelve-step and other self-help groups, where the concept of service is central to recovery. One study conducted by researchers at Brown University Medical School reinforces what Bill W. (one of the two founding members of AA) already knew. Alcoholics involved in helping others achieve sobriety are significantly less likely to relapse themselves.[31] Of those in the study who helped others, forty percent stayed sober in the first year following treatment. Of those who didn't help others, only twenty-two percent remained sober in that following year.

Likewise, studies conducted on patients experiencing chronic pain from illnesses such as multiple sclerosis have shown that when patients support other patients in pain through doing things like phone check-ins their own pain decreases and their moods improve. Depression and anxiety decrease and self-confidence and hope increase.[32] Similar studies on patients with other conditions show the same results. Patients who help others reap both physical and mental rewards.

These benefits extend all the way to lifespan. Older adults in one study were divided between those who volunteered (in any capacity) for more than or less than four hours a week. Those who volunteered more than four hours a week saw a reduction of mortality of up to forty-four percent.[33] We can actually live longer by serving others.

In contrast to the notion that we have evolved to be selfish creatures in a world where only the most adaptable survive, giving and compassion seem to be linked to our evolutionary brain. Studies using functional magnetic resonance imaging show that when subjects give, whether in time or money, parts of the primitive brain associated with the pleasures of sex and eating light up. Researchers see this as a biological explanation for what is called "helper's high," that warm and fuzzy feeling we get when we do something good. But it's not just a warm and fuzzy feeling; that high has real measurable benefits. The helper's high was first described by Allan Luks, who studied thousands of volunteers across the United States and found that people consistently noticed an improvement in their health when they started volunteering.[34]

More evidence shows that compassion is biologically rooted in the brain. University of Wisconsin psychologist Jack Nitschke studied a group of new mothers. When the new moms looked at pictures of their babies, portions of their brains associated with positive emotions lit up, and they reported feelings of compassion. In an unrelated study, Joshua Greene and Jonathan Cohen of Princeton University scanned the brains of people when they were engaged in contemplating harm being done to others. What they found was that a similar part of the brain that lit up with the new moms also lit up with these subjects. The same part of the brain associated with compassion fires when we look at our own offspring and when we witness perfect strangers being harmed.[35]

Further studies have indicated that when we're able to help someone in distress, brain activity in the caudate nucleus and anterior cingulate are stimulated. These are located in the same region of the brain that turns on when we receive rewards or experience pleasure. What all these studies indicate is that compassion is hardwired into our brains. And it brings us pleasure. As Thich Nhat Hanh teaches, "[a] person without compassion cannot be a happy person."[36]

I have yoga students who'll protest that they can't spend their whole lives serving others. They think this is an ideal they can't achieve, and in truth they aren't sure they'd really want to even if they could. These students have received a healthy amount of training in the school of self-care, and they are not altogether wrong. The teachings on karma yoga, renunciation, and selfless service certainly don't mean we have to sacrifice our own best interest. Yoga teaches us that when we serve our own ego, we don't actually find the happiness we're seeking. The real path to happiness is serving the interests of the Divine Self. The Divine Self thrives in connection and living in harmony with others, on compassion and generosity. But as Stephen G. Post, a professor of bioethics at Case Western Reserve University School of Medicine and the president of The Institute for Research on Unlimited Love, says, "just as excessive focus on self may be unhealthy, an excessive focus on others may be unhealthy as well."[37]

Dr. Post makes the case that although a certain amount of service is beneficial for all, we can also become overwhelmed, and the benefit of serving begins to diminish as this happens. For example, those caring for chronically ill loved ones can become exhausted and so drained that they feel they have nothing left to give. Activists who work with unrelenting suffering in war zones, or activists for whom the issue of animal suffering seems insurmountable, can also understandably lose the helper's high after seeing too much misery. We can be overcome by our own compassion and drain ourselves in our giving. So, Dr. Post says, we must take time to care for ourselves to ensure we don't burn out.[38]

As we've seen, this advice is consistent with spiritual teachings. I had the opportunity to visit Thich Nhat Hanh's home monastery in the South of France during the summer of 2014, before Thay, as his students call him, had a stroke. During the summer months, Plum Village monastery opens up for public retreats. Before his stroke, Thay would conduct three Dharma talks a week and one question-and-answer session during these retreats. When you're with him, you know you are in the presence of an enlightened being. You can see the peace and compassion in his eyes, in each gentle step he takes, and in the way he smiles. You can feel it being called forth from your own being. On the morning of the first Q&A session, I went to the front of the meditation hall and sat next to him. We listened to three sounds of the bell and then I asked him my question: "How can I best help the animals who suffer so much as a result of human activity?"

Thay had many wise and inspiring words to offer me, but the first thing he said, as he looked at me with the eyes of the most profound understanding and compassion, was, "You cannot drown in your own sorrow." He went on to tell me I needed to maintain a spiritual practice in order to touch the seeds of happiness and joy within myself and the world, so I'd have the energy to continue to help.

❈

There are so many ways we can serve. We can serve our families every day by paying attention and listening to them. Then, from the understanding that comes from that attention, we can serve them more in myriad ways—from cooking wholesome food with love, to holding their hand as we sit at the doctor's office to learn of the test results, or taking the dog on a daily walk.

Yoga teaches us to serve in the way that is natural for us. As Lord Krishna tells Arjuna, "It is better to strive in one's own dharma than to succeed in the dharma of another. Nothing is ever lost in following one's own dharma, but competition in another's dharma breeds fear and insecurity."[39]

The real message of all the spiritual teachings is not only to serve the few creatures we know as families and friends, but to serve all beings in whatever capacity we can: "Love thy neighbor as thyself" (Mark 12:31). Some may serve best by becoming doctors or lawyers championing the rights of those who cannot defend themselves. Some may serve best by making music that brings people peace or cooking wholesome foods that benefit the human body, while respecting Earth and other animals. We might spend time with Alzheimer's patients at a local senior center or help build a water sanitation system in an African village. Krishna's message is that we don't need to serve in the way others do. We can do everything in the spirit of service. We can dedicate all of our actions to the well-being of others. The message is that in whatever way we can, let us open our hearts to others, dedicate all actions to the welfare of others, and then follow the unchartered, unique, and perfect paths that unfold from our own hearts. ❈

5

A Practical Manual for Living One Step at a Time

Depending on where we start, the idea of wellness can be overwhelming. There's so much information to absorb. If we try to take it all on at once, we may feel it's too much, which can be self-defeating. My own personal path toward increasing wellness, health, and wholeness has been very gradual and organic. I didn't set out to get healthy. My own healthy habits have evolved over a very long time. I grew up eating more junk food than anyone I've ever known. I quite literally ate fast food every day of my life from the age of perhaps four to about eighteen. I ate meat and dairy at every meal until my first attempt at vegetarianism at the age of sixteen. But I was inspired by my aversion to animal cruelty rather than any interest whatsoever in my own health, so even my early forays into vegetarianism were filled with French fries, potato chips, milkshakes, tater tots, cheesy pizzas, and red licorice. But it was a start.

I knew nothing about nutrition then and didn't care to know. My diet was terrible, and I felt like garbage. Doctors told me I had irritable bowel syndrome (IBS) and prescribed medicine that didn't work. Practically everyone I knew told me I needed meat to be healthy, so when I felt sick, I thought maybe they were right.

After about two years of being vegetarian, I convinced myself that the government had eliminated animal cruelty. In my very optimistic and naïve mind, I thought if I knew about the cruelty, then the government did, too, and in the world

I believed I lived in, my government wouldn't allow that kind of mass suffering to continue. That wasn't a world or a reality I was prepared to accept. I went back to eating meat but gave it up again every couple of years when something happened to stir my conscience. I wavered in this way for decades.

I also spent most of my youth getting into trouble with a big, bold, capital T. Rather than playing sports or doing anything remotely healthy or physically active, I started smoking cigarettes at age ten and pot at eleven. I drank throughout my adolescence, consumed large amounts of various drugs, and generally lived an unhealthy, delinquent life until, gradually and naturally, the bad habits began to drop away and things began to change in my twenties. Self-loathing helped me lose my taste for drugs by the end of my teens, and vanity prompted me to start exercising at about the same time.

A decade later, I finally found the motivation to give up animal products for good. It was not my own health that motivated me this time either, but an under-cover video of a fur farm, after which I pledged I would never in any way again take part in the immense body of animal suffering. Knowing how much I'd struggled in the past with maintaining a vegetarian diet, I wanted to make sure I wouldn't sabotage myself again by becoming malnourished through a diet of French fries and Twizzlers. So I started to research nutrition.

I was amazed to discover how perfect a plant-based diet is when done right—and actually how simple "right" is when it's understood. I started making changes to my diet slowly. Instead of eating pesto pasta with processed spaghetti, I mixed half whole-wheat spaghetti noodles with the white noodles, until over time I lost my taste for the processed, refined stuff and came to prefer the healthier whole-grain version. I scrutinized labels to avoid the most toxic ingredients like hydrogenated oils, in addition to the myriad animal products food manufacturers sneak into our processed foods. (For example, the ingredient carmine, which is commonly used in fruit juices, candies, frozen popsicles, and colored pastas, is actually ground-up insects!)

After reading *The China Study*, I began trying to eat a whole foods, plant-based diet, adding in as many new grains, beans, and vegetables I could find and realizing how many edible and delicious plants I'd overlooked until then. I became more aware of the difference between processed foods and whole foods. Gradually, my eating habits grew healthier, and I started to feel better than I ever had before. The IBS that plagued me throughout my twenties disappeared.

But some habits die hard. I only quit smoking at the age of thirty-five when I went to India and learned to breathe without inhaling through a cigarette. It was also in India that I learned patience. Whether we were learning asana or philosophy or standing in line for food, my teachers would repeat the refrain "slowly, slowly." Yes, everything comes in time. Everything we do builds on what we've done before. Changes happen when the time is right. Awakening happens gradually. It's like when we're waking up in the morning after a long, hard sleep: we wake up progressively, the way the sun rises or the room lightens as it does.

We must take things at our own pace—start where we are and keep learning and make the changes that come naturally when the learning sinks in enough to get us to adopt the changes we know will help us. This is why it's so important to approach ourselves holistically. We can try to change our habits through suppression and shame, but this isn't included in any recipe for long-term wellness. Change will come when we develop awareness of our habits and triggers, and the ways we sabotage ourselves. Change will come with patience and steady practice.

Santosha or "Progress, not Perfection"

A mantra I often have to remind myself of is "progress, not perfection." It's important to know what the goal is and where the target is, so that we can focus in that direction. But it's equally important to stay in the present, and to practice patience and understanding with ourselves along the way. The second of Patanjali's niyamas is *santosha*, which means contentment: *samtosad anuttamah sukha labhah*, "By contentment, supreme joy is gained."[1] We are where we are. If we try to be somewhere else, we get into trouble. If we can see the lessons available in our current circumstances and find peace in the present moment, we lay the foundation for ultimate happiness.

When I was first practicing yoga, I would see yogis popping into headstands next to me in class, and I always thought I was physically incapable of ever standing on my head. I told myself I was just not built for headstands, and I remember being afraid that I'd develop a blood clot and literally die if I even tried. Then the day came where I popped up, too. The headstand has many benefits, including awakening the crown chakra and revitalizing the entire mind and body. But the main benefit was my epiphany that I could accomplish many other things if I could overcome the self-limiting concepts that held me back from even trying.

It's also true that if yoga has any goal, it's not about what the final physical posture looks like. It's not about touching our heads to our knees or our bellies to the floor, or standing on our head or in any other posture. Our goal is to be fully present in the here and now, to move in and out of postures (and the rest of our lives) with mindfulness, awareness, and ideally, without ego. "The path to the temple is the temple," as some wise, anonymous Buddhist once said.

On the path to peace, dissatisfaction is a classic obstacle. When we're constantly comparing ourselves to others (what they have, what they've accomplished, what they look or feel like, or whatever it is), we're bound to feel unsatisfied. The practice of santosha is to be aware of all the conditions we have for happiness *right now*. We fail to appreciate what we have until it's gone; we fail to appreciate our eyesight until we begin to experience macular degeneration; we fail to appreciate the dog until he's diagnosed with cancer; we fail to appreciate the lack of pain in our joints until we develop rheumatoid arthritis. The Buddha taught that we have wholesome, unwholesome, and neutral seeds in our consciousness.[2] When we are mindful, we learn how to cultivate the wholesome or positive seeds, to stop watering the unwholesome or negative ones, and to turn the neutral seeds into positive ones. We do this every time we become grateful for something we've taken for granted.

We are often inclined to compare ourselves to those we see as having more than us. This is so much of what popular culture is based on: the ads and movies, the tabloids and celebrity talk shows. Everywhere we go, it seems, we're bombarded with images of people living some kind of good life, if material abundance and excess are the measure. This is when it's critical we apply the teachings in our daily lives. When we look deeply, we can see that while there are people living in gigantic mansions, with the resources to spend a fortune on every imaginable luxury, millions of people in the world are starving to death who'd literally give an arm to have what we take for granted. If we and our families are safe and healthy, with food to eat and a roof over our heads, we have more than enough to be happy. Our happiness does not depend on obtaining anything more. It depends on seeing what's already here.

What's more, we learn that our happiness depends on our internal state anyway, not on our external conditions. When we're connected to the Divine Self, with our minds clear and our hearts open, we'll know we have enough and will be content with what we have. We'll be grateful for every breath of life and every moment we can share with our loved ones. We'll cherish every day we're able to extend some kindness into the world, for every sunset we see and every meal we enjoy.

Whereas santosha teaches us to recognize the many gifts that fill our lives, and can help us to connect with joy in every moment, I must stress that it doesn't imply complacency or settling for something that's not good for us or for someone else. It definitely doesn't mean we give up on ourselves or the world. It means having patience in our journey, realizing that both personal and sociopolitical growth and progress happen over time. Our journeys are more of a marathon than a sprint, and we need to pace ourselves or we will burn out. Santosha means doing the best we can right now with enough patience to sustain us as we move forward toward more peace and more love. Santosha saves us from the trap of believing that happiness awaits us in some future time, when some condition has manifested. It tells us happiness is possible in this very moment. It means we put one foot in front of the other and breathe mindfully as we continue to walk along our path, responding to what calls to us, and appreciating the journey on the way.

Each Day a New Beginning

How we begin each morning has a real impact on the way the day will unfold. When we wake up, our minds can be all over the place depending on how we slept, what we dreamed, and what we have planned for the day ahead. It's helpful to recalibrate the mind when we wake up and go to bed, bookending our days with aspirations and reflections. If instead of racing out of bed and blindly rushing into our routine we can create the habit of pausing and centering ourselves, it will pay off throughout the day. Ultimately, as our lives are really no more than a collection of our days, it will transform the content of our lives.

Oftentimes, though the alarm goes off and we open our eyes and get out of bed, we continue to sleepwalk through the day. In order to really wake up, we need more than an alarm. We need a practice that washes away the fog of the mind and reveals the light of the heart. If meditation is not (yet) your practice at this time of day, the following four practices can help you do this.

1. Make a Gratitude List (At Least a Mental One)

Start the day by reminding yourself of all the things you can be thankful for. If you're blessed to have a companion with whom you wake up—a partner, a spouse, a dog or cat—just look over and realize this blessing. You might think of all the people in the world who don't have a warm bed or companionship. We take the basics for granted the most, such as being physically able to get out of bed. If we were too sick to get up, we'd be keenly aware of our misfortune. On the flip side, we are usually completely unconscious of the greatest blessings of life, such as health, physical safety, a home, and food to eat.

If we can begin each day by reminding ourselves of these gifts, we won't allow the precious moments of our short lives to slip by unnoticed until it's too late to recapture them. We can transform even the irritations of life into cherished moments. Through eyes filled with gratitude, we come to appreciate the textures of our lives and each other in a new and invigorating way, and transform a life that might have felt mundane or oppressive into one that resonates with the sacred.

2. Breathe

Before getting out of bed, take a moment to find your breath and deepen it. With each breath, we come into a new and fresh moment. With each day, we begin anew. In Plato's *Cratylus*, the Greek philosopher Heraclitus says, "No man ever steps into the same river twice, for he is not the same man, and it is not the same river." Breathe into the present moment on this new day and feel the freedom that comes when we allow this truth.

3. Find Your Heart

As we pause and breathe, we can draw the breath into the heart and reconnect with the sensations there. The vow of the bodhisattva is to commit every day to achieving enlightenment for the sake of all beings. This can translate into our own daily lives as a commitment to stay awake, to be mindful, and to work on releasing ourselves from our ego-based neurosis for the sake of all living beings, including ourselves.

When we reconnect with the heart, we begin to reconnect with our fundamental nature, our Divine Self. If we start each day from a place of tenderness in the heart, we open ourselves to every joy and sweetness it may offer us. When we start the day rooted in the true Self, we set our course with the confidence and strength of having a full wind in our sails. This is what we need to help carry us through the day so we can to make it meaningful and well lived.

4. Set an Intention for the Day

Starting the day with some simple intentions can help us stay on course throughout the day. When we begin to get lost, don't know the next right move or right thing to say, or just find ourselves feeling uncomfortable in any given situation, we can remember our intentions and use them to keep ourselves in check, to re-center.

a. **Commit yourself to being mindful through the day.** This means examining your thoughts and emotions as they arise, watching for the *kleshas*, or mental obstacles, which include our fears, ego-clinging, and everything else that arises when we've lost touch with our Divine Self. Such a process of losing touch is the avidya, or fundamental ignorance from which all other obstacles arise, and is known in the modern world as "issues" or neurosis. When we see them coming up, we can work with them by pausing and watching ourselves. We can use whatever arises as an opportunity for growth and self-awareness.

b. **Set an intention to use your good fortune for the benefit of the world.** Each day, we can commit to doing our best to live in a way that our actions cause no harm to any other being (including ourselves) and, ideally, are of some benefit to at least one other being.

At night, we can reflect on how closely our thoughts, words, and actions throughout the day accorded with the intentions we set. The point is not to judge or reprimand ourselves for where we may have strayed but to learn from all of our experiences. As we doze off, we do so in the act of recommitting ourselves to our intentions to be mindful, to keep our hearts open, and to be of service to all in need. In this way, we begin weaving these aspirations into our deepest layers of consciousness. As the days pass, we begin to notice they are transforming our lives.

Sadhana—Our Practice

Sadhana is a Sanskrit word referring to the range of spiritual practices that help us stay connected to the Divine Self within: that help us stay anchored in peace. We are Divine. We are pure. We are the Buddha. We are the lotus. But we have this sort of congenital amnesia and forget who we really are. A spiritual practice can be anything that helps us remember our Divine nature; that helps us to realize our true, authentic selves.

My friend David, who teaches yoga in Rehoboth Beach, Maryland, mentioned to me several years ago his concept of a "toolbox," which has been helpful for me ever since. Each of us has our own metaphorical toolbox, filled with the things we need to wake us up and help us reconnect, feel centered, alive, and whole. We need to draw from that toolbox and grab the tool that's called for at any given moment.

From a yogic framework, traditional sadhana may include meditation, pranayama, yogasana, mantra, scriptural study, and karma yoga, for example. Our personal practices may include these and anything else that helps us find our peace and our hearts. To our list of sadhana we might add kayaking or hiking in nature, attending church, journaling, spending time with or otherwise talking with family, being with animals or by ourselves, etc.

It can be helpful to make a list with three columns, writing down all the things we need to do on a daily, weekly, or occasional basis to feel whole, at peace, and centered. We need to pay attention and figure out what these are, and then make the time to do them.

Nature's Temple

For many, nature provides a perfect temple in which to connect with the Divine Self. In nature, we can find the peace and calm in which we're able to notice this eternal presence within. In her temple, surrounded by the elements of earth, air, fire, and water, the Divine within is instinctively called forth to commune with the Divine that surrounds us. Nature's abundance, fecundity, grace, and ease surpass and still the mind and speak directly to the soul.

According to the biophilia hypothesis of biologist E. O. Wilson, human beings have an innate instinct to connect emotionally with nature.[3] The term *biophilia* was originally coined by German sociologist Erich Fromm as "love of life or living systems."[4] *Philia* is the Greek word for "love," the opposite of a phobia, and according to Wilson, we've got it bad for nature.

Wilson asserts that the human affinity for the environment is deeply rooted in our biology. This connection is not just with forests, mountains, and beaches but with animals as well. An increasing body of scientific research supports the healing connection between humans and nonhuman animals. In a study conducted over thirty years ago, researchers found that heart-attack patients with companion animals lived longer than those who didn't. And it's been shown that simply petting one's own dog reduces blood pressure. More recent research indicates that spending time with animals increases our body's own production of oxytocin, the same hormone our bodies release when we fall in love and which aids in healing and new cell growth.[5] This information not only reinforces our strong bond with animals but also the mind–body connection, as well as our inborn ability to heal ourselves.

From a Vedic perspective, our connection with nature runs even deeper, as we are seen as sharing the same fabric of existence with the natural world. The Divine is believed to manifest itself in animals as much as in human beings, and the Divine essence is believed to permeate all life from rivers to mountains, grassland and forest, sky and stars. The essential view is captured in a conversation between the sage Uddalaka and his son Shvetaketu in the *Chandogya Upanishad*, one of the oldest of the ancient Indian scriptures, dating back to the seventh or eighth century B.C.E.:

> As by knowing one lump of clay, dear one,
> We come to know all things made out of clay—
> That they differ only in name and form,
> While the stuff of which all are made is clay;
>
> As by knowing one gold nugget, dear one,
> We come to know all things made out of gold—
> That they differ only in name and form,
> While the stuff of which all are made is gold;
>
> As by knowing one tool of iron, dear one,
> We come to know all things made out of iron—
> That they differ only in name and form,
> While the stuff of which all are made is iron—
>
> So through spiritual wisdom, dear one,
> We come to know that all of life is one.

In the beginning was only Being,
One without a second.
Out of himself he brought forth the cosmos
And entered into everything in it.
There is nothing that does not come from him.
Of everything he is the inmost Self.
He is the truth; he is the Self supreme.
You are that, Shvetaketu; you are that. [. . .]

As bees suck nectar from many a flower
And make their honey one, so that no drop
Can say, "I am from this flower or that,"
All creatures, though one, know not they are that One.
There is nothing that does not come from him.
Of everything he is the inmost Self.
He is the truth; he is the Self supreme.
You are that, Shvetaketu; you are that.

As the rivers flowing east and west
Merge in the sea and become one with it,
Forgetting they were ever separate streams,
So do all creatures lose their separateness
When they merge at last into pure Being.
There is nothing that does not come from him.
Of everything he is the inmost Self.
He is the truth; he is the Self supreme.
You are that, Shvetaketu; you are that![6]

In our modern world, it's so easy to forget that we are that. We forget that we're a part of nature, biological beings constructed out of the same substances as all other creatures. We're made of atoms and cells recycled from the beginning of time. We have this idea that we aren't a part of nature, but that she's merely here for us to exploit and to subdue. This idea is so fallacious it ranks with other mental conditions like schizophrenia or delusional disorder. We don't see that as we exploit nature, we exploit ourselves.

According to the World Wildlife Fund (WWF), between forty-six and fifty-eight thousand square miles of forest are destroyed annually[7]—equivalent to losing thirty-six football fields every minute. We clear forests for agricultural uses—primarily to graze our cattle or raise crops to feed them, as well as to make way for massive oil pipelines and logging. We might as well take up smoking, because the forests are the lungs of the planet, absorbing harmful CO_2 gases and producing the oxygen we need to survive.

For those of us living in the suburbs or rural areas, our relationship with nature is often more accurately defined as a battle than a communion. In 2011, 13.7 million people, or six percent of the U.S. population sixteen years old and older, went hunting, and more than thirty-three million Americans over sixteen went fishing.[8] We douse our weeds with herbicides, spray our plants with fungicides, and bathe our gardens in pesticides. In 2011, the total amount of U.S. cropland certified as organic was 0.8 percent, less than one percent! The remaining ninety-nine percent of U.S. crop and other farmland was saturated by chemicals.[9]

Our connection with nature is both metaphysical and very tangible. The damage we do to the environment, we do to ourselves. We've enslaved billions of animals and deprived them of any semblance of a natural life. We're poisoning the water we swim in and the water we drink. We pollute the air we breathe. On a societal level, we need to reevaluate our relationship with the environment in a fundamental way.

On a personal level, reestablishing our connection is of primary importance. As with all practices, we must begin with ourselves. The personal healing involved in reconnecting with nature is not separate from planetary healing. It takes a shift in us as individuals to move society toward balance. We find our own balance, and in doing so we bring a part of the world back into balance. We may only be a drop in the ocean; but as Rumi reminds us, the ocean is also in the drop.

In the West, we tend to view ourselves as separate from nature. In sharp contrast to the passage from the *Chandogya Upanishad* quoted above, the Judeo-Christian tradition in Genesis offers another framework for understanding the ideal relationship between humanity and our environment. In 1:24–26 (NIV), God proclaims:

> And God said, "Let the land produce living creatures according to their kinds: the livestock, the creatures that move along the ground, and the wild animals, each according to its kind." And it was so. God made the wild animals according to their kinds, the livestock according to their kinds, and all the creatures that move along the ground according to their kinds. And God saw that it was good.
>
> Then God said, "Let us make mankind in our image, in our likeness, so that they may rule over the fish in the sea and the birds in the sky, over the livestock and all the wild animals, and over all the creatures that move along the ground."

In his book *Dominion: The Power of Man, the Suffering of Animals, and the Call to Mercy*, Matthew Scully makes the argument that because God gave humanity dominion over the animals, we have a duty to care for them and we're doing an abominable job.[10] But it's a problematic paradigm to begin with. The argument is that because we're the overlords, we should be just and merciful. This is analogous to keeping slaves in comfortable conditions. It's a paradigm based on oppression and inequality.

In contrast, Eastern philosophy is deeply rooted in a reverence for Mother Nature. For millennia, this wisdom has shaped the way in which Eastern cultures view the human–nature bond. Dr. David Frawley writes, "The ancient Seers knew that all of Nature is part of the individual, since we all are created from, exist in, and return to nature. Individuality is thus a very temporary condition that can flourish only with Nature's assistance, not Her enmity."[11]

In order to bring ourselves to a point of health, we must reestablish our own connection with nature: our own and that which surrounds us. We can be mindful of how our actions impact the environment: from the foods we eat to the cars we drive (or even better don't drive), avoiding chemicals on our own lawns and in the beauty and cleaning products we use.

We also benefit tremendously from spending at least some time in nature every day. In fact, we *must* be outside. To receive adequate amounts of vitamin D, which is so essential to preventing cancer and maintaining strong bones, we need to be in the sunshine at least thirty minutes a day. People heal faster and experience elevated moods when exposed to light.[12]

Our bodies and minds are affected by nature whether we know it or not. When we develop a personal relationship with nature, we notice the changing of the seasons as different birdcalls sound or different flower buds emerge and fade away, as leaves fall or grasses burst through the hard ground. We aren't merely spectators at this perpetually fluctuating show. As the fall winds blow, the hairs on our arms rise. We breathe in the crisp air; our blood vessels constrict. Our moods reflect these changing cycles in the environment.

Beyond the measurable physical benefits of nature, we know we feel something when we stand at the shore and inhale the sea air; walk through the woods chasing curious dragonflies; stand in the forest at dawn and glimpse the aptly named morning glory with its delicate, white tubular flower and deep purple center; or spot the toad waking from his nightly hibernation, still too slow to escape had we been a real predator. Moments such as these restore our true state of dignity and confidence. They offer strength beyond ego—the strength and dignity that come when we understand in a very deep, experiential way that we're a part of the Divine and connected to everything. They restore our innate integrity and faith in ourselves.

The connection we feel with nature offers hints about our connection with the universe and helps us release ego and the ideas of separateness that have allowed our species to damage the environment and devastate so many other species, both farmed and wild. It's easy to forget our kinship with nature until we are in it.

Habits

> [T]o be driven by appetite alone is slavery, and obedience to the law one has prescribed to oneself is liberty.—**Jean-Jacques Rousseau**[13]

For most of us, our lives are just a collection of habits: some "positive" some "negative." The more we repeat a behavior, reaction, or thought, the more ingrained that behavior, reaction, or thought becomes. With each repetition we create a memory, something of a mental groove that becomes deeper and deeper every time we repeat the behavior. Modern brain science tells us this is why beating addiction gets harder over time. In Sanskrit, these grooves or mental impressions are called samskaras. They are formed not just by what we do but by how we view the world, relate to other people, and think. They manifest as our habitual reactions and perceptions— the filter through which we view and experience the world. They make up our conditioning.

As we continually repeat the same responses, over time we begin to identify ourselves with them and create a self-identity around them. In effect, we believe we *are* our habits, so we think change is not possible. Patanjali tells us this false identification with our habits is one of the major obstacles (kleshas) most of us confront on our paths to wholeness and well-being:

> *Avidyasmita raga dvesabhinivesah klesah*: Ignorance, egoism, attachment, hatred, and clinging to bodily life are the five obstacles.[14]

> *Anityasuci duhkhanatmasu nitya suci sukhatmakhatir avidya*: Ignorance is regarding the impermanent as permanent, the impure as pure, the painful as pleasant, and the non-Self as the Self.[15]

The first major obstacle, ignorance, is the root of all the others. We identify with our habits and the ever-changing qualities and circumstances of our lives, taking these to be who we are. We forget that in truth we are the pure, Divine Self, the spacious awareness that lies at our foundation, the basic goodness that we are. We begin to see ourselves as this collection of impermanent qualities and habits. We cling to ego and our self-conception as a separate and distinct entity. Consequently, we forget that true peace and happiness lie within and start looking for these outside of ourselves. We seek pleasure (*raga*) and avoid pain (*duhkha*)—and miscalculate what actually brings either.

For example, say having forgotten my true nature (*avidya*), I cling to my ego (*asmita*) and identify myself as a single forty-five-year-old man with depression, diabetes, and a genetic predisposition to an early heart attack. I tell myself "I am" lonely, and in my quest to obtain happiness and avoid suffering, I spend evenings at a strip club drinking myself into a stupor and giving away all my money to women who don't really care about me and who are suffering in their own right. I wake up in the morning feeling ill and filled with self-loathing, depression, and loneliness. So, I go back to the bar night after night and continue the cycle.

As Patanjali explains, we see our impermanent, non-Self qualities as permanent, forgetting entirely the qualities of the Divine Self within: the peace, joy, happiness, and love that have always been in our hearts and are still there now. We confuse what is pleasant and what is painful, believing that drinking or drugging or shopping (or whatever our personal escape is) will ease our suffering, when the truth is, in the long run, it only amplifies it.

As we begin to look at our habits through the lens of mindfulness, we see that we're not our habits. We are the Divine Self, always pure, always whole and complete. We have only forgotten. We begin to realize we can change our habits once we see they aren't us. All things of this world are impermanent. We can choose to cultivate habits that bring us pain and suffering, or we can choose to cultivate habits that bring us peace and help us return to the state of balance that is our true nature.

Thich Nhat Hanh says, "Because suffering is impermanent, that is why we can transform it. Because happiness is impermanent, that is why we have to nourish it."[16]

One of the most empowering and liberating teachings yoga offers is that we can do things differently: things we never thought we were capable of. We can be the people we want to be. Breaking habits begins with awareness. We want to cultivate awareness of the habits themselves and the ideas we put on top of those habits, the self-limiting beliefs that surround our habits, like "I'm not smart enough," "I'm not attractive enough," "I'm not strong enough," or whatever our own habitual thought patterns are telling us.

Once we see these patterns, we can begin to work with them. There is a Zen story about a man on a horse that demonstrates the force of our habit energies. The man comes charging into town on his horse one day, and it appears he is going somewhere very important. Another man rides over and asks, "What's going on? Where are you going so fast?" The first man replies, "I don't know. Ask the horse."[17] Our habits are like energetic horses that race us around town and we go along for the ride. We have to pause and pay attention, observe what we're doing and what habits we're engaging in that cause us to suffer. Once we become aware, we can begin to do something about them.

If I went to a doctor with an amorphous pain in my abdominal area but couldn't be any more specific about its location or my discomfort, the doctor probably wouldn't be able to help me. But if she ordered a diagnostic test like a CT scan and could determine I had kidney stones, she could treat me. Similarly, if I can identify what my habit energy or pattern is, I can work on changing it.

Through the filter of our Western minds, we usually view practices such as diet and exercise in a very superficial and compartmentalized way. Often, we deprive ourselves of what we like and force ourselves to do what we dislike to achieve some idea of physical fitness or limited idea of health. Then we head into battle with ourselves. We try to force "good" habits on ourselves and suppress the "bad." This struggle is self-sabotaging.

In one of my favorite Buddhist stories, as told by Buddhist nun Pema Chödrön, Milarepa returns to his Himalayan cave after gathering firewood or the nettles that constitute his ascetic diet and finds his cave populated by demons. They're eating his food, sleeping in his bed, and generally making themselves at home. Milarepa is very troubled by these demons. But he's a devout and experienced yogi, so he sits down very calmly and tries to talk to them about the Dharma. He explains the Buddha's teachings on non-duality and how we're all one, as well as on compassion and the major Buddhist teachings. But the demons don't budge. They simply continue what they were doing.

At this point, Milarepa grows frustrated and impatient and begins to scream at the demons to get out of his cave. That just makes them angry. Their eyes grow red, their fangs grow longer, and they laugh and gnash their teeth at him like Maurice Sendak's wild things. Apparently seeing the futility in his struggle, Milarepa surrenders. He sits on the floor and in effect says, "OK, stay if you want to. I don't care." At that point, all of them leave, except one—a really nasty demon. This time, instead of using more force, Milarepa surrenders more deeply. He walks over to the demon and climbs right into his mouth—saying, writes Pema Chödrön, "Just eat me up if you want to." At that point—poof!—the demon vanishes.[18]

As a society, we're so entrenched in the model of struggle that we just keep prodding the demons. We need to learn nonresistance. Nonresistance doesn't mean we simply give up and in to our basest tendencies—go without bathing, stop cutting our toenails, eat potato chips, and watch TV on the couch all day. That's what makes this path a bit tricky. We walk the razor's edge between struggling and succumbing.

In yoga or our other mindfulness practices, we learn to watch our minds and the thoughts as they arise. Instead of suppressing them, we learn to look at them with mindfulness and without judgment and then stop chasing them. When we do so, they begin to dissolve. If we suppress them, they rise up with renewed vigor. If we indulge them, they carry us off like helpless prisoners with our hands and ankles bound. So we do something else. We watch. We breathe. We let go. We move on.

As we incorporate the teachings into our lives, we can apply them with this same gentleness. If an urge arises to eat a juicy cheeseburger, for instance, we have three choices: we can fight the urge; we can succumb; or we can watch it, accepting that it's there, and then let it drift off. This is the nature of all things: they float in and float away. We can witness this for ourselves when we begin to watch the thoughts that arise in our minds.

It's as if we were sitting in a room at the top of a tall building, looking out a window. A bunch of red balloons suddenly sails across our view from left to right. We watch them travel across the sky. We might wonder where they came from. We could go down the elevator and run into the street and chase after them, as they bob among the buildings and out across the river, eventually perhaps landing in a tree. Or we might sit in our comfortable chair and watch them float across the sky until they disappear. Either way, they would come from who knows where and disappear just as mysteriously. The same is often true of our own thoughts, emotions, and desires. Their origin is unknown and they dissolve, if we let them.

Releasing the struggle associated with compulsions also becomes much easier as our awareness increases. As it does, an authentic compassion for ourselves arises, which prompts us to want to take care of ourselves. Further, as our sense of connectedness with others increases, and we see how our actions affect not just ourselves but others as well, we find the strength to do things differently. For as egotistical as we may seem to be as a species, our own selfish, personal desires have far less energy than our altruistic ones. When we do things just for ourselves or rather for our ego-selves, we may find we are weak. In contrast, we find unexpected and tremendous strength when motivated by love.

For example, I have been lactose intolerant my whole life. Since childhood, whenever I ate dairy products I became sick with a range of nasty gastrointestinal issues. I'd take pills with my food to try to reduce the effects, and sometimes I'd decide not to order a pizza because I wanted to avoid discomfort. But I craved cheese so much I never even really considered giving it up despite my discomfort. However, once I learned and finally accepted the truth about how dairy cows and their calves are treated, I gave up dairy and never looked back.

If we're trying to purify the body for superficial, ego-based reasons, we may not find the discipline required to see through on our intentions. When we begin to link the practices together and see that our own health is part of a much bigger picture—connected with our families, friends, society, other species, and the planet—something shifts. We discover the strength that had eluded us thus far.

The Four Noble Truths

As we work on transforming our habit energies, the Buddha's teaching of the Four Noble Truths can be of great benefit. The Buddha summed it up when he said, "I teach only suffering and the end of suffering. That's all I teach." We can use these Four Noble Truths to transcend our own suffering and habits. They are as follows:

> The truth of suffering (*duhkha*)
> The truth of the origin of suffering (*samudāya*)
> The truth of the cessation of suffering (*nirodha*)
> The truth of the path to the cessation of suffering (*magga*)

The first truth is the realization that there's a problem. The second truth is to see and identify what's causing that problem. This involves reflection and often taking responsibility, but it also provides us with hope, because if we are responsible for our suffering, we have the power to change it. The third truth is seeing that if we stop doing these things, we can change. Finally, the fourth truth tells us that there's a path that leads to the end of suffering. That path is the Eightfold Path, which consists of right view, right intention, right speech, right action, right livelihood, right effort, right mindfulness, and right concentration.

If, for example, we suffer because of the foods we eat, we can practice mindfulness, become aware of what we're doing and how it's causing us and others harm.

Then, in order to know that we can stop doing what we're doing and can change, we have to look for alternatives, and understand how the alternatives can lead us out of suffering. For example, if we have clogged arteries and suffer because we have heart pain and fear we're going to die, we can see how the food we eat is causing the arteries to be clogged. We realize that if we eat a plant-based diet, our heart condition will improve. Then we put our insight into action. Empowered with all the knowledge we have, we run to the market, raid the produce section, and come home and cook up something that's so good it puts an end to our suffering.

We know our food can be toxic or can be healthful. The Buddha taught that, similarly, what we ingest through our senses and our minds can similarly be toxic or healthful: from the television we watch, to the people we spend time with, to the images we choose to look at on the Internet, and everything else we come into contact with. The Buddha taught us to consume only what nourishes happiness and peace and to stop ingesting that which makes us feel toxic—whether it's food, certain conversations, people, or anything else.

For example, if we watch a violent television show, we may notice that we feel fearful or angry and that those emotions linger after we've turned the TV off. Again, we could apply the teaching of the Four Noble Truths. First, we'd notice that we're having disturbing feelings. Second, we'd identify that they are coming from the sort of television we're watching. Third, we'd realize we could stop watching these types of program. Fourth, we'd take action by changing our behavior. Maybe we change the channel and watch something that helps us reconnect with right view, like a program about the cosmos that reminds us of the miracle of life. Or maybe we turn off the television entirely and walk the dog or do anything else that helps us water the seeds of mindfulness, the seeds of awareness, and compassion within ourselves.

As we progress on the path of mindfulness, we see our own destructive behavior more clearly. Then maybe we get stuck for a while. We see what we're doing. We know what we need to do to feel better, but we just can't seem to do it. Not yet. This is key. Just because we aren't able to let something go immediately doesn't mean we won't be able to at some point. Seeing the habit has tremendous power to free us from it. With nonjudgmental awareness of these habits and the continued application of our practices, the destructive habits do eventually fall away. The more mindful we are of our habits and how they harm us or others, and the more we see how we can do things differently, the closer we come to actually doing things differently.

Another helpful tool Patanjali gives us for changing our destructive habits is *pratipaksha bhavana*, or replacing the disturbing force with a positive one. He states: *vitarkabadhane pratipaksha bhavanam*. "When disturbed by negative thoughts, opposite [positive] ones should be thought of. This is pratipaksha bhavana."[19]

Sometimes, this way of thinking can help us get past that block. The idea is that once we become aware of the thought, pattern, or behavior disturbing our peace, we can replace it with its opposite. If, every night before bed, I splurge on ice cream, which exacerbates my borderline diabetes and makes me feel terrible about myself, I might simply replace the ice cream with a healthier alternative, like a smoothie made with fruit and some raw cocoa. Who knows? Eventually, maybe I'll let that go, too.

The more aware we are of our patterns and the more we understand them, the easier it will be to transform them. Once we really understand what the underlying emotional need is, we can find more appropriate, effective ways of "feeding" the need. So, when the craving for ice cream, or television, or wine, or whatever our thing is, comes up, if we can pause and mindfully breathe into the feelings in the heart, stomach, or whole body—without labeling, just feeling the sensation—we might be able to identify what the *real* longing is. Of course, sometimes we may actually be hungry, like when we haven't eaten in many hours. As Sigmund Freud said, sometimes a cigar is just a cigar! But when dealing with destructive habits, we need to look deeply enough that we come to understand what the real longing is.

An urge arises to grab the ice cream container. After pausing and reflecting, I realize I'm trying to mask a sense of dissatisfaction. On further investigation, I realize that dissatisfaction is really sadness over having had a fight with my mother earlier that day. Result: I can skip the ice cream and call Mom. Or if I comprehend that the feeling in my heart is isolation and loneliness, I might reach out to a friend or loved one. Or I might go to my cushion and meditate, reconnecting with the Divine within, the source of all fullness.

It's important to know what it is that helps us reconnect with that Divine Self and what brings us joy. This is what our toolbox is for. When swapping unhealthy habits for healthy ones, we can dig into our toolboxes. It's very helpful to establish new routines and rituals as we work on changing habits. Establishing routine practices and habits in all areas of our lives will help them become second nature. The more established we become in our spiritual practices, the more they'll help us take those actions that lead us away from suffering. The more we live our lives based on ahimsa, satya, and the other ethical principles, and in awareness and service, the easier it becomes to make the choices that end our own suffering.

Discover Your Sankalpa

Sankalpa is a Sanskrit word that translates as something like "intention" or "resolution." It differs from what we think of as a New Year's resolution like "I will quit smoking." A sankalpa is a statement of fulfillment of the heart's deepest longing. Sankalpa is often used in conjunction with a *yoga nidra* practice, which is a form of deep, guided meditation.

The first step in developing a sankalpa is to tune in to that inner voice and listen. When we're still and the mind is quiet, we can begin to hear what the heart deeply longs for. The next step is to imagine we have that thing. For example, if my heart yearned for peace—true, deep peace—I'd imagine what it would feel like to be utterly filled with peace: with no worries, fear, or anxiety. The sankalpa is a statement that grows out of that feeling of satisfied longing. A sankalpa, therefore, is usually phrased positively and in the present, something like "I am . . ." or "I feel. . . ." So, maybe, "I am peace," or "I feel the peace that is flowing through my heart at all times," or "I am filled with peace." If your heart's deepest longing is to feel really healthy, you might just say "I am healthy."

Sankalpa is based on reconnecting with the deep truth that we are always full and whole. Our fears and experiences, learned behaviors, traumas, disappointments, etc. lead us to believe/fear we are lacking and incomplete in some way. When we work with sankalpa we come into the heart and return to the fullness we've forgotten is our true nature. We can begin incorporating our sankalpa into our lives like a mantra, returning to it as we meditate or at the beginning of a yoga class. We might use it before we go to bed, repeating it silently to ourselves as we fall asleep. As we do, we plant that intention at the deepest layers of consciousness.

By becoming very clear with ourselves about what we want, we give ourselves focus. We plant a seed and nurture it until it grows to be a strong oak. In the *Dhammapada*, the Buddha taught that everything begins with a thought: "Our life is shaped by our mind; we become what we think. Suffering follows an evil thought as the wheels of a cart follow the oxen that draw it. Our life is shaped by our mind; we become what we think. Joy follows a pure thought like a shadow that never leaves."[20] So let us choose and cultivate our thoughts with care and intention.

Changing Food Habits

Almost everyone engages in some form of emotional eating at times. Our associations with food go back to the first meal we took, possibly at our mother's breast. We were hungry and she gave us food in the most intimate, loving way imaginable. It's no wonder that we look to food not just for nutritional sustenance but for something much deeper, much more emotional. Unfortunately, after weaning, food doesn't come packaged in quite that much devotion and love again. It can give us pleasure and sustenance, and there's nothing wrong with either. But we get into trouble when we look for it to provide something it can't give. This is true of all external sources of pleasure and happiness. There's nothing wrong with enjoying our food, relationships, or our careers. We can enjoy the range of our experiences, but if we look to them for everlasting peace and happiness, to feel whole, loved, calm, and happy, we're bound to be disappointed.

The key to breaking the cycle of emotional eating (or any other unhealthy addictive cycle for that matter) is awareness. When we notice we're getting pulled into this cycle, we begin by pausing and finding our breath. Ask yourself: *What am I really craving? Is it food? Or is it something deeper?* Breathe right into the feeling. Just identifying the true feeling will help break that habitual cycle. When we realize what we crave is love, for example, it becomes clear we won't get it from fried chicken, even if it's made from tofu! When we want love, we need to turn to a source that can give us love—maybe a friend, family member, pet, or the Divine within our own hearts. We shouldn't expect deeply ingrained long-term habits to fall away on their own overnight. However, seeing our habits and identifying the underlying needs provide the necessary foundation for us as we work on getting unstuck.

It's also important not to confuse discipline with deprivation. For some, the ascetic route might work, but for most of us deprivation is a setup for failure. This is why traditional diets usually don't work. When we're eating a whole foods, plant-based diet, we don't have to deprive ourselves. But as with all things, we need to pace ourselves. At some point, your taste buds may change enough that anything other than the natural sugars found in fruits will be unappealing, but if you're not quite there yet, it can be helpful to focus on replacing the worst sweets with healthier alternatives—like switching from processed, store-bought cookies to homemade whole-grain cookies, or eating small quantities of dark vegan ethically sourced chocolate for dessert at night and aiming for chocolate with a high cocoa content.

As you work toward new routines, consider incorporating the following suggestions:

- Establish set meal times and try to stick with them as much as possible.
- Sit down to eat.
- Focus on slowing down the whole process of eating to heighten awareness of underlying emotional patterns. Focus on deepening and slowing the breath before eating.
- Take a few deep breaths before you eat anything.
- Consider saying a prayer before you eat, or repeating an affirmation or mantra.
- Make your own healthy alternatives of the unhealthy comfort foods that might be sabotaging you. For example, bake your own sweets. You'll get the benefit of knowing what is in your food, and home-

Relapse Prevention

Stock your kitchen with healthy foods. Food relapses are bound to happen when we are unprepared, and that's when emotional and unhealthy eating happens. Avoid this by always having something in the kitchen you can grab and heat up or cook quickly. For example, I always try to keep the following items stocked in my house: *(contd.)*

Cashews, almonds, walnuts

Nut butters

Trail mix

Fresh and dried fruit

Frozen fruit for smoothies

Nut milks (soy, almond)

Organic spices

Dried and canned beans (garbanzo beans, black beans, lentils)

Tofu

Tempeh

Ground flaxseeds (add to smoothies, replaces eggs in baking)

Miso paste

Maple syrup or molasses

Tea bags

Granola or other whole-grain cereals

Whole grains (brown or wild rice, quinoa, whole-wheat spaghetti)

Extra virgin olive oil

Vinegar (apple cider, red, balsamic, rice)

Vegetarian deli meats (bologna, turkey, ham)*

Veggie burgers

Veggie crumbles (Smart or Boca)

Earth Balance or other vegan margarine

Tamari (or soy sauce is fine, too)

Vegetable bouillon cubes

In addition:

- Keep a few vegan frozen meals in your freezer, as well some healthy soups in the pantry.
- Whenever you make a big pot of soup or stew, freeze a portion.
- Keep frozen veggies in the freezer to eat in a pinch.

If you do choose to eat something unhealthy, avoid the cycle of guilt by forgiving yourself and having compassion for that part of you that is looking for happiness.

* Eventually you would ideally wean yourself from the processed "mock" meats and cheeses, but they are very helpful as we transition.

baked goods are always going to be healthier than the store-bought versions. When baking at home, use raw sugar instead of processed, or maple syrup to sweeten. Also, you can use whole-grain flours, plus fruits, vegetables (like carrots or zucchini), or nuts, which will make those baked goods nutritious.

- Pay attention to what kinds of foods you gravitate toward, and seek out healthy versions. These days, everything, or at least a recipe for everything, is available on the web.

How to Eat!

General Principles

In transitioning to a more harmonious, clean diet, focus on what you're adding to your diet and your life, rather than what you're giving up. Transitioning to a plant-based diet turns out to be more about what you add than what you avoid. Letting go of what we're comfortable with is never easy, whether it's a relationship, job, hairstyle, or familiar foods. (A bird in the hand, and all that.) Once we let go of that thing we cling to despite the pain it causes us, we open ourselves to the possibility of receiving something better. In this case, that means better health and skin, a healthier weight, a clearer conscience, and a bounty of new delicious whole foods to discover.

As a general rule, we want to eat foods that come straight from the earth without processing. Lightly cooking our foods is the best way to make them digestible without killing off nutrients. Many people believe that eating food raw is the healthiest option, but it doesn't matter how nutritional the food itself is if we can't absorb the nutrients properly. As Ayurveda teaches us, we need to listen to our bodies. We want to eat as many whole, unprocessed foods as possible. Whether they're raw or lightly cooked will depend on our individual constitution.

When we transition to a plant-based diet, we want to experiment with new ingredients. Go to the produce section of your local supermarket; even better, visit the farmers market and try anything new that draws your attention. CSAs are also a great way to discover new foods and eat what's in season because your farm share will be of whatever is growing locally right now.

Don't worry that you're going to have to give up everything you love to eat. You can modify many of your favorite dishes to make them vegan. Replace eggs with ground flaxseeds in baking so you can continue to enjoy your favorite baked goods. Use raw cashew cream to make dishes creamy. Use nut milks instead of dairy milks. Go online and find recipes for vegan versions of your favorite foods. There's a vegan version for just about everything! More importantly, watch your consciousness expand, as you open yourself up to a new way of thinking about food and how to build nutrient-dense and delicious plant-based meals.

For most of us, it will be helpful to keep things simple at the beginning to avoid becoming overwhelmed. Depending on what you're used to eating and your general enjoyment of cooking, transitioning to a whole foods, plant-based diet may seem complicated. There are certainly a lot of complicated recipes out there! Most of us are busy and need to balance eating the best foods we can with those busy schedules, so simple recipes may be optimal.

Also, spending a few hours over the weekend prepping for the week will make putting meals together during the week a lot easier. Preparing soups in advance and keeping washed and chopped fresh veggies (as well as frozen) stocked in the house should make it relatively easy to stick to healthy dinners. Try incorporating some vegetables and legumes (beans) into your soups. Serve with a side of raw or steamed vegetables, plus some kind of whole grain like quinoa, wild rice, or whole-grain bread—all of which can be prepared in advance.

Generally, aim to eat a plant-strong diet. If you're not ready to go the whole way, that's OK. But aim to reduce animal products and increase plant-based foods as much as possible. If you're used to eating meat with every meal, try giving up meat on Mondays, then add Tuesday, Wednesday, and so on. If you've already given up meat but have a hard time letting go of dairy, try a dairyless Monday, with the same idea of experimenting in a way that's not overwhelming.

Changing practices, especially those as deeply ingrained as our eating habits, isn't easy. But once we take the first step, it gets exponentially easier with time. In short order, we feel more energy; our digestive tracts work more efficiently; our waistlines begin to shrink; and we like ourselves better. A real spiritual pleasure arises when we find ourselves living in harmony with ourselves and with our precious world.

The Conscious Plate

To synthesize and simplify all the information we now have about right diet, it can be helpful to build your daily meals around a modified version of the USDA new food pyramid, or what is now called MyPlate.[21] If we could imagine all the food we eat in a given day arranged on one plate, we'd want to aim for a quarter whole grains, a quarter plant-based protein sources, a quarter fruits, and a quarter vegetables. Following are a few ideas of what foods this model might include.

Whole Grains

The recommended intake for whole grains is six to eleven servings per day.* Examples of foods in the whole grains group include:

Quinoa	Bulgur	Unprocessed cereals
Barley	Whole-grain bread	(oats, cream of wheat,
Oats	Whole-grain rice	muesli, puffed whole-
Millet	Whole-grain pasta	grain cereal)

* It's important to stress that the grains are of maximum benefit when unprocessed and whole. (If the first ingredient says "enriched flour" it is not a whole grain.)

Legumes, Nuts, Soy, and Other Protein Sources

This group includes sources of protein and calcium, with the recommended daily consumption of five to eight servings. These foods include:

Cooked peas, beans (black, kidney, cannellini, adzuki, turtle, lima, black-eyed, garbanzo, and the list goes on and on!), and lentils	Fortified nut milks
	Seeds
	Meat analogs (vegan meat substitutes, such as meatless burger patties)
Nuts or nut butters	
Tofu, tempeh	Hummus or tahini

Vegetables

The vegetable group includes fresh, canned, or frozen veggies. We should aim for *at least* four servings of vegetables each day. Some highly nutritious suggestions for vegetable choices are:

Broccoli	Swiss chard	Butternut Squash
Cauliflower	Spinach	Sweet potatoes
Kale	Carrots	Leeks
Collard Greens	Zucchini	Cabbage

Fruits

Two or more servings of fruit are recommended each day. There are a number of easy ways to get your fruit servings in, including:

- Fresh fruits (apples, oranges, berries, etc.)
- Canned or frozen fruit
- Dried fruit
- Fruit juice or smoothies (but avoid smoothies filled with syrups, ice cream, and milk, and stick with homemade smoothies made with fresh or frozen fruit, juice, nut milks, baby spinach leaves, ground flaxseed, etc.)

Fats and Oils

Although we want to avoid saturated fats (such as those coming from animal products) and other added fats in foods, many naturally occurring fats are beneficial to our health. Two servings of these good plant-based fats are recommended daily. Good fats and oils can be found in:

Olive or canola oils	Flaxseeds and flaxseed oil
Nuts and nut butters	Hempseed or hemp oil
Green or black olives	Walnuts
Avocados	

While we are aiming for progress and not perfection, there are some pretty toxic, disease-causing ingredients that we want to eliminate entirely from the diet. Besides meat and dairy, these include:

- White sugar
- High fructose corn sugar
- Aspartame and other artificial sweeteners
- Saturated fats (primarily from animal products including meat and dairy)

- Hydrogenated oils
- All artificial food dyes
- White flour (we really want to eliminate all refined grains that include white flour, like breads, pastas, cakes, etc.)

Juicing and Fasting

Fiber is an essential component of a healthy diet. It helps detoxify the body and keeps the digestive tract working. But it fills us up. When we extract the juice from fruits and vegetables, we isolate their vitamins and other nutrients without the fiber. We can consume a higher density of nutrients when we're not getting too full from the fiber. I might be able to eat two cups of broccoli in one sitting but I could probably juice five times that amount. Mostly, though, we want to juice only vegetables, not fruit, as we end up with too high a concentration of sugar when we juice fruits—other than lemons, which are highly alkalinizing and not too sweet. To make juice more palatable, we can include sweet beets and just a little apple. Adding juice to a whole foods diet is a great way to obtain all the benefits of the whole foods while supplementing the diet with these added nutrients.

Juicing can also be part of a healthy fast. Ayurveda recommends fasting for a twenty-four-hour period each week, consuming nothing but vegetable juices, herbal teas, and water or lemon water during this time. As healthy as our food may be, it takes a lot of work and energy for the body to process and digest food. Giving the body a rest from time to time can help us feel lighter, more clear-headed, and more energetic, and generally promote overall health. A fast can also be especially detoxifying and healing whenever we have overeaten.

It's no accident that juicing and fasting come at the end of this book. While both can be a healthy component of wellness, as I began the book by saying, there is no single physical practice that alone can bring us into a state of holistic wellness. True health comes from finding harmony in mind, body, and spirit—harmony within and with the world. ❁

ॐ
Conclusion

Since the beginning of recorded history, human beings have struggled to understand our world, to grasp the meaning of our lives. Sages and philosophers have sought to understand the world through concepts and categories. In Ancient Greece, intellectual giants like Plato and Aristotle introduced the approach of grouping objects and classifying them based on their similar properties. It's hard to imagine how we'd function without some kind of systematic conceptual approach to life. The problem is we've mistaken the "approach," or tool, for the Ultimate Reality. Even the Buddha said, "My teaching is like a finger pointing to the moon. Do not mistake the finger for the moon."[1]

Because we live in a world of categories and pointing fingers, the idea that all things are interconnected or that "we are all one" can seem a little far out. But even if the idea of the unity of all things seems esoteric to us, the fact becomes tangible when we look at how inextricably interrelated our food choices are with the well-being of billions of nonhuman animals, humans on the other side of the world, our own health, and the planet itself. Our food choices have an impact that goes far beyond this assembly of particles we call "ourselves." What we eat affects all life on this planet. The standard American diet of cheeseburgers and ice cream that clogs arteries and causes cancer is responsible for the mass suffering of billions of living beings and a leading cause of world hunger and our environmental crisis.

A plant-based diet can reverse our own illnesses and lead us to health. It will prevent an ocean of suffering and heal the planet. Our choices determine whether we all thrive or we all suffer. The diet best for the planet is best for human health.

Once we've touched the truth of who we truly are, if we live in a way that helps us stay connected to this truth—applying ahimsa, satya, asteya, aparigraha, the Four Immeasurable Minds of Love, and the other teachings into our lives—the path to purity, peace and health, and a good life unfold before us. When we're in harmony with ourselves, we come into harmony with the world. This leads us to health in all areas of our being, from our physical bodies to our emotional and spiritual selves, and ultimately extends to all other beings and the world. Consequently, as all things are connected, in our quest for personal purity, we could end up not only saving ourselves, but saving the world.

> May all the pain of every living being
> Be wholly scattered and destroyed.
> For all those ailing in the world,
> Until their every sickness has been healed,
> May I myself become for them
> The doctor, nurse, and medicine itself.
> My body, thus, and all my goods besides,
> And all my merits gained and to be gained,
> I give them all away withholding nothing
> To bring about the benefit of beings.
> May I be a guard for those who are protectorless,
> A guide for those who journey on the road.
> For those who wish to go across the water,
> May I be a boat, a raft, a bridge.
> And now as long as space endures,
> As long as there are beings to be found,
> May I continue likewise to remain,
> To drive away the sorrows of the world
> —**Shantideva,** *The Way of the Bodhisattva* ❁

Notes

Chapter 1: Yoga as a System of Purification

1. See *The Yoga Sutras of Patanjali* translated by Swami Satchidananda. Yogaville: Integral Yoga Publications, 2010 (1978), p. 127.

2. Quoted in *The Yoga of Spiritual Devotion* translated by Prem Prakash. Rochester, Vt.: Inner Traditions, 1998, pp. 77–81.

3. Thich Nhat Hanh. *Awakening of the Heart: Essential Buddhist Sutras and Commentaries.* Berkeley: Parallax Press, 2012, pp. 499–500.

4. See "Environmental Impacts" by Pesticide Action Network North America (PANNA). <http://www.panna.org/resources/environmental-impacts>.

5. "Behind Mass Die-Offs, Pesticides Lurk as Culprit," by Sonia Shah. *Environment 360*, January 7, 2010 <http://e360.yale.edu/feature/behind_mass_die_offs_pesticides_lurk_as_culprit/2228/>.

6. Thich Nhat Hanh. "The Five Mindfulness Trainings" <http://plumvillage.org/mindfulness-practice/the-5-mindfulness-trainings/>.

7. *The Bhagavad Gita* translated by Eknath Easwaran. Petaluma, Calif.: Nilgiri Press, 2010 (1985). All quotations from the *Gita* are from this edition.

8. Swami Satchidananda, *Yoga Sutras* (1:14).

9. Shantideva. *The Way of the Bodhisattva.* Boston: Shambhala, 2006, p. 127.

10. See Thich Nhat Hanh, *The Heart of the Buddha's Teaching.* New York: Broadway Books, 1998, pp. 31–37.

11. Ibid., p. 33.

12. John Robbins. "Any Connection Between What You Eat and Your Spiritual Evolution?" The Food Revolution Network, March 24, 2014 <http://foodrevolution.

org/blog/any-connection-between-what-you-eat-and-your-spiritual-evolution/>.

13. See *Upanishads* translated by Eknath Easwaran. Petaluma, Calif.: Nilgiri Press, 2009 (1987), p. 80.

14. Cited in Hanh, *Heart of the Buddha's Teaching*, pp. 179–180.

15. See *Cartesian Reflections: Essays on Descartes's Philosophy* by John Cottingham. New York: Oxford University Press, 2008.

16. See "Pig Video Arcades Critique Life in the Pen," by Miguel Helft, *Wired*, June 6, 1997 <http://www.wired.com/1997/06/pig-video-arcades-critique-life-in-the-pen/>.

17. The Humane Society of the United States. "More about Pigs: The Underestimated Animal," 2009 <http://www.humanesociety.org/animals/pigs/pigs_more.html>.

18. Quoted in *The Oxford Handbook of Animal Ethics* edited by Tom L. Beauchamp and R. G. Frey. Oxford: Oxford University Press, 2011, p. 235.

19. Quoted in *Animals and World Religions* by Lisa Kemmerer. Oxford: Oxford University Press, 2012, p. 96.

20. Norm Phelps. *The Great Compassion: Buddhism and Animal Rights.* New York: Lantern Books, 2004, p. 47.

21. Chögyam Trungpa Rinpoche. *Shambhala: The Sacred Path of the Warrior.* Boston: Shambhala, reprint edition, 2007, pp. 33–34.

22. See *Big Book of Alcoholics Anonymous*, Chapter 5, "How It Works."

23. Swami Satchidananda, *Yoga Sutras*, p. 131.

24. For a nuanced interpretation of Gandhi's statement, see "Gandhi on Providence and Greed" by Y. P. Anand and Mark Lindley, Academia.edu <http://www.academia.edu/303042/Gandhi_on_providence_and_greed>.

25. Pew Charitable Trusts and Johns Hopkins Bloomberg School of Public Health. *Putting Meat on the Table: Industrial Farm Animal Production in America*, 2008 <http://www.ncifap.org/_images/pcifapfin.pdf>.

26. Humane Society of the United States. "Farm Animal Statistics: Slaughter Totals" <http://www.humanesociety.org/news/resources/research/stats_slaughter_totals.html>.

27. Animal Legal Defense Fund. "Farmed Animals and the Law" <http://aldf.org/resources/advocating-for-animals/farmed-animals-and-the-law/>.

28. Farm Forward. "Ending Factory Farming." Farm Forward's calculation is based

on U.S. Department of Agriculture, *2012 Census of Agriculture*, June 2014 <http://farmforward.com/ending-factory-farming/>.

29. Animal Welfare Institute. "Animal Welfare Act" <https://awionline.org/content/animal-welfare-act>.

30. Animal Welfare Institute. "During Transport" <https://awionline.org/content/during-transport>.

31. Ibid.

32. Paul Solotaroff. "In the Belly of the Beast," *Rolling Stone*, December 10, 2013 <http://www.rollingstone.com/feature/belly-beast-meat-factory-farms-animal-activists>.

33. Ibid.

34. "Humane Methods of Slaughter Act: Weaknesses in USDA Enforcement." Statement of Lisa Shames, Director, Natural Resources and Environment, GAO-10-487T, March 4, 2010 <http://www.gao.gov/assets/130/124119.pdf>.

35. For more on the inhumane conditions of animals on factory farms, see *Farm Sanctuary: Changing Hearts and Minds About Animals and Food* by Gene Baur. New York: Touchstone, 2008.

36. Bruce Friedrich. *Huffington Post*, "The Cruelest of all Factory Farm Products: Eggs from Caged Hens," January 14, 2013 <http://www.huffingtonpost.com/bruce-friedrich/eggs-from-caged-hens_b_2458525.html>.

37. Humane Society International. "An HSI Report: The Welfare of Animals in the Egg Industry," updated March 2011 <http://www.hsi.org/assets/pdfs/welfare_of_animals_in_the_egg.pdf >.

38. Kimberly Kindy. "USDA Plan to Speed Up Poultry-Processing Lines Could Increase Risk of Bird Abuse," *Washington Post*, October 29, 2013. <https://www.washingtonpost.com/politics/usda-plan-to-speed-up-poultry-processing-lines-could-increase-risk-of-bird-abuse/2013/10/29/aeeffe1e-3b2e-11e3-b6a9-da62c264f40e_story.html>.

39. United Poultry Concerns. "Forced Molting," 2015 <http://www.upc-online.org/molting>.

40. Sean Poulter. "The Disturbing Conveyor Belt of Death Where Male Chicks Are Picked Off and Killed So You Can Have Fresh Eggs," *Daily Mail*, November 4, 2010 <http://www.dailymail.co.uk/news/article-1326168/Secret-footage-shows-millions-British-chicks-killed-year.html>.

41. ASPCA. "The Truth About Chicken" <http://truthaboutchicken.org/>.

42. ASPCA. "A Closer Look at Animals on Factory Farms" <https://www.aspca.org/animal-cruelty/factory-farms/animals-factory-farms>.

43. See Nick Cooney. *Veganomics: The Surprising Science on What Motivates Vegetarians, from the Breakfast Table to the Bedroom.* New York: Lantern Books, 2014, p. 8.

44. Theodore Xenophon Barber. *The Human Nature of Birds: A Scientific Discovery with Startling Implications.* New York: St. Martin's Press, 1993.

45. See "IQ Tests Suggest Pigs Are Smart as Dogs, Chimps," by Jennifer Viegas, Discovery News, June 11, 2015 <http://news.discovery.com/animals/iq-tests-suggest-pigs-are-smart-as-dogs-chimps-150611.htm>.

46. For more on our different attitudes toward species see *Why We Love Dogs, Eat Pigs, and Wear Cows: An Introduction to Carnism* by Melanie Joy. San Francisco: Conari Press, 2009.

47. J. Vansickle. "Quality Assurance Program Launched," *National Hog Farmer,* February 15, 2002 <http://nationalhogfarmer.com/mag/farming_quality_assurance_program>.

48. Grass-fed beef has its own problems and is arguably even more environmentally destructive, as more land and other resources are required to raise the animals. Most of the destruction of the rainforest can be attributed to grass-fed beef production.

49. PBS, *Frontline.* "Modern Meat," Interview with Michael Pollan <http://www.pbs.org/wgbh/pages/frontline/shows/meat/interviews/pollan.html>.

50. Ibid.

51. See National Resources Defense Council. "Antibiotic Use in Livestock Going Up, Up, Up," by Avinash Kar, April 10, 2015 <http://switchboard.nrdc.org/blogs/akar/antibiotic_use_in_meat_and_pou.html>. For more on antibiotic use, see Pew Charitable Trusts. "Overuse of Antibiotics in Food Animal Production: Science Fact Sheet," May 2014 <http://www.pewtrusts.org/~/media/Assets/2014/06/Overuse_Science_Backgrounder_v3.pdf>.

52. To see a feedlot, visit Compassion in World Farming. "Battery Beef: Welcome to the Feedlot," by Philip Lymbery, November 21, 2014 <http://www.philiplymbery.com/2014/11/battery-beef-welcome-to-the-feedlot/>. See also *Farmageddon: The True Cost of Cheap Meat* by Philip Lymbery and Isabel Oakeshott. London: Bloomsbury, 2014.

53. David S. Turk. "Overview of Cattle Laws," Animal Legal and Historical Center,

Michigan State University College of Law, 2007 <https://www.animallaw.info/article/overview-cattle-laws>.

54. For more on dairy cows' experience, see "Milk of Human Kindness Denied to Dairy Cows," by James McWilliams, *Forbes*, October 25, 2013 <http://www.forbes.com/sites/jamesmcwilliams/2013/10/25/milk-of-human-kindness-denied-to-dairy-cows/>.

55. USDA. "Veal from Farm to Table" <http://www.fsis.usda.gov/wps/portal/fsis/topics/food-safety-education/get-answers/food-safety-fact-sheets/meat-preparation/veal-from-farm-to-table/ct_index>.

56. Cooney, *Veganomics*, p. 5.

57. Culum Brown. "Not Just a Pretty Face," *New Scientist* 2451 (2004): 42–43.

58. Jonathan Balcombe. *Pleasurable Kingdom: Animals and the Nature of Feeling Good.* New York: Macmillan, 2006, p. 188.

59. Animal Welfare Institute. "Fish Farming" <https://awionline.org/content/fish-farming>.

60. Cooney, *Veganomics*, p. 8.

61. For more on fish and their welfare, visit Fish Feel <http://www.fishfeel.org/>.

62. See Cooney, *Veganomics*, p. 8.

63. FAO. *Livestock's Long Shadow: Environmental Issues and Options*, 2006 <ftp://ftp.fao.org/docrep/fao/010/a0701e/a0701e00.pdf>.

64. NASA. "Earth's Fidgeting Climate," October 20, 2000 <http://science.nasa.gov/science-news/science-at-nasa/2000/ast20oct_1/>. See also "The Consequences of Climate Change" <http://climate.nasa.gov/effects/>.

65. Just how much is a contested figure. For a relatively cautious assessment, visit UNEP. "Growing Greenhouse Gas Emissions Due to Meat Production," October 2012 <http://na.unep.net/geas/getuneppagewitharticleidscript.php?article_id=92>.

66. FAO. "Key Facts and Findings" <http://www.fao.org/news/story/en/item/197623/icode/>. This number is FAO's revision of their estimation of eighteen percent (more than all transportation emissions combined) in *Livestock's Long Shadow*.

67. Robert Goodland and Jeff Anhang. "Livestock and Climate Change: What If the Key Actors in Climate Change Are . . . Cows, Pigs, and Chickens?" *World Watch* 22, no. 6, November/December 2009. pp. 10–19 <http://www.worldwatch.org/files/pdf/Livestock%20and%20Climate%20Change.pdf>.

68. FAO. "Livestock a Major Threat to Environment; Remedies Urgently Needed." November 29, 2006. <http://www.fao.org/newsroom/en/news/2006/1000448>.

69. "Is Meat Sustainable?" *World Watch* 17, no. 4, July/August 2004 <http://www. worldwatch.org/node/549>.

70. See Water.org. "Water-related Disease Facts." <http://water.org/water-crisis/disease-facts/> and Water.org. "Water Facts & Sanitation Facts." <http://water.org/water-crisis/water-sanitation-facts/>.

71. National Geographic. "Freshwater Crisis" <http://environment.nationalgeographic. com/environment/freshwater/freshwater-crisis/>.

72. H. J. I. Marlow, W. K. Hayes, S. Soret et al. "Diet and the Environment: Does What You Eat Matter?" *American Journal of Clinical Nutrition* 89, no. 5 (2009): 1699S–1703S. doi: 10.3945/ajcn.2009.26736Z.

73. Michael F. Jacobson. "More and Cleaner Water." In *Six Arguments for a Greener Diet: How a More Plant-Based Diet Could Save Your Health and the Environment.* Washington, D.C.: Center for Science in the Public Interest, 2006 <http://www. cspinet.org/EatingGreen/pdf/arguments4.pdf>.

74. Jenny Barchfield. "Experts: Nearly 1 Billion Hungry People in World," *Capital Press*, May 6, 2009 <http://www.klamathbasincrisis.org/agriculture/articles/09/ experts1billionhungry050609.htm>.

75. Alastair Bland. "Is the Livestock Industry Destroying the Planet?" Smithsonian.com, August 1, 2012 <http://www.smithsonianmag.com/travel/is-the-livestock-industry-destroying-the-planet-11308007/?no-ist>.

76. "Our Food Our Future: Making a Difference with Every Bite—The Power of the Fork!" EarthSave International <http://www.earthsave.org/pdf/ofof2006.pdf>.

77. Philip Thornton, Mario Herrero, and Polly Ericksen. "Livestock and Climate Change." *Livestock Exchange Issue Brief* 3 (November 2011) <https://cgspace.cgiar. org/bitstream/handle/10568/10601/IssueBrief3.pdf>.

78. *World Watch*, "Is Meat Sustainable?"

79. FAO. "Livestock a Major Threat to Environment."

80. Ibid.

81. *Cowspiracy: The Sustainability Secret.* Produced by Kip Anderson and Keegan Kuhn, 2014.

82. Minority Staff of the U.S. Senate Committee on Agriculture, Nutrition, and Forestry, "Animal Waste Pollution in America: An Emerging National Problem." Report compiled for Senator Tom Harkin, December 1997, p. 11.

83. Natural Resources Defense Council (NRDC). "Facts about Pollution from Livestock Farms," updated February 21, 2013 <http://www.nrdc.org/water/pollution/ffarms.asp>.

84. David Wallinga, M.D., Institute for Agriculture and Trade Policy. "Concentrated Animal Feeding Operations: Health Risks from Air Pollution," November 1, 2004 <http://www.iatp.org/files/421_2_37388.pdf>.

85. NRDC. "Facts about Pollution."

86. See "Overfished and Under-protected: Oceans on the Brink of Catastrophic Collapse," Tom Levitt, CNN, March 27, 2013 <http://www.cnn.com/2013/03/22/world/oceans-overfishing-climate-change/>.

87. C. Picone and D. Van Tassel. "Agriculture and Biodiversity Loss: Industrial Agriculture" in *Life on Earth: An Encyclopedia of Biodiversity, Ecology, and Evolution* edited by Niles Eldredge. ABC-CLIO, 2002, pp. 99–105.

88. Jeffery S. Pettis, Elinor M. Lichtenberg, Michael Andree, et al. "Crop Pollination Exposes Honey Bees to Pesticides Which Alters Their Susceptibility to the Gut Pathogen *Nosema ceranae*," *PLoS ONE* 8, no. 7 (July 24, 2013), doi: 10.1371/journal.pone.0070182.

Chapter 2: Right Diet as a Way of Life: Beyond the Cleanse

1. Quoted from T. Colin Campbell, Ph.D. and Thomas M. Campbell II. *The China Study: The Most Comprehensive Study of Nutrition Ever Conducted and the Startling Implications for Diet, Weight Loss, and Long-term Health.* Dallas: BenBella Books, 2006.

2. Quoted in *The Food Revolution: How Your Diet Can Help Save Your Life and Our World* by John Robbins. San Francisco: Conari Press, 2011, p. 47.

3. Quoted in Robbins, *The Food Revolution*, p. 51. Brackets in *The Food Revolution*.

4. Campbell and Campbell, *The China Study*, p. 33.

5. Ibid.

6. John Robbins. *Healthy at 100.* New York: Ballantine Books, 2007.

7. EarthSave. "Food Choices and Your Health" <http://www.earthsave.org/healthy.htm>.

8. Michael Greger, M.D. "Is Milk Good for Our Bones?" *Nutrition Facts* 23 (March 16, 2015) <http://nutritionfacts.org/video/is-milk-good-for-our-bones>.

9. Jack Norris, R.D. "Calcium and Vitamin D," Vegan Health, updated October 2013 <http://www.veganhealth.org/articles/bones>.

10. Jack Norris, R.D. "Iron," Vegan Health, updated June 2013 <http://www.veganhealth.org/articles/iron>.

11. Jack Norris, R.D. "What Every Vegan Should Know about Vitamin B_{12}," Vegan Health <http://www.veganhealth.org/articles/everyvegan>.

12. For a relatively balanced assessment, visit Harvard School of Public Health. "Vitamins" <http://www.hsph.harvard.edu/nutritionsource/what-should-you-eat/vitamins/>.

13. See Physicians Committee for Responsible Medicine, "The Nutrition Rainbow" <http://www.pcrm.org/sites/default/files/pdfs/health/Nutrition_Rainbow.pdf> and Julie Garden-Robinson, Ph.D., L.R.D. "What Color Is Your Food?" North Dakota State University, reviewed May 2011 <https://www.ag.ndsu.edu/pubs/yf/foods/fn595.pdf>.

14. Non-GMO Project. "What Is GMO?: Agricultural Crops That Have a Risk of Being GMO" <http://www.nongmoproject.org/learn-more/what-is-gmo/>.

15. UNEP, International Assessment of Agricultural Knowledge, Science and Technology for Development, *Agriculture at a Crossroads*, Global Report. Washington, D.C.: Island Press, 2009 <http://www.unep.org/dewa/agassessment/reports/IAASTD/EN/Agriculture%20at%20a%20Crossroads_Global%20Report%20(English).pdf>.

16. Felicity Carus. "UN Urges Global Move to Meat and Dairy-free Diet," *Guardian*, June 2, 2010 <http://www.theguardian.com/environment/2010/jun/02/un-report-meat-free-diet>.

17. A. Coleman-Jensen, M. Nord, M. Andrews, et al. "Household Food Security in the United States in 2011." USDA, September 2012 <http://www.ers.usda.gov/media/884525/err141.pdf>.

18. UNEP. "Food Waste: The Facts" <http://www.worldfooddayusa.org/food_waste_the_facts>.

19. Charles M. Benbrook. "Impacts of Genetically Engineered Crops on Pesticide Use in the U.S.—the First Sixteen Years." *Environmental Sciences Europe* 24, no. 24 (2012), doi: 10.1186/2190-4715-24-24.

20. A. Samsel and S. Seneff. "Glyphosate's Suppression of Cytochrome P450 Enzymes and Amino Acid Biosynthesis by the Gut Microbiome: Pathways to Modern Diseases." *Entropy* 15, no. 4 (2013): 1416–1463, doi: 10.3390/e15041416.

21. Kevin Bonham. "Allergic to Science: Proteins and Allergens in Our Genetically Engineered Food." *Scientific American*, May 30, 2013 <http://blogs.scientificamerican. com/guest-blog/allergic-to-science-proteins-and-allergens-in-our-genetically-engineered-food/>.

22. Judy A. Carman, Howard R. Vlieger, Larry J. Ver Steeg, et al. "A Long-Term Toxicology Study on Pigs Fed a Combined Genetically Modified (GM) Soy and GM Maize Diet." *Journal of Organic Systems* 8, no. 1 (2013): 38–54, <http://gmojudycarman.org/ wp-content/uploads/2013/06/The-Full-Paper.pdf>.

23. For more on chlorpyrifos, see PANNA. "Chlorpyrifos" <http://www.panna.org/ resources/chlorpyrifos-0>; CDC. "Fourth National Report on Human Exposure to Environmental Chemicals, 2009." pp. 135–139 <http://www.cdc.gov/exposurereport/ pdf/fourthreport.pdf>; and EPA. "Chlorpyrifos." updated October 30, 2015 <http:// www2.epa.gov/ingredients-used-pesticide-products/chlorpyrifos>.

24. Brenda Eskenazi, et al. "The Pine River Statement: Human Health Consequences of DDT Use," *Environmental Health Prospect* 117, no. 9 (September 2009): 1359–1367, doi: 10.1289/ehp.11748.

25. Eric Schlosser. "Access to Good, Healthy Food Should Be a Basic Human Right," *The Atlantic*, February 22, 2012 <http://www.theatlantic.com/health/archive/2012/02/ access-to-good-healthy-food-should-be-a-basic-human-right/253349/>.

26. Environmental Working Group, "Dirty Dozen" <http://www.ewg.org/foodnews/ dirty_dozen_list.php>.

27. Environmental Working Group, "Clean Fifteen" <http://www.ewg.org/foodnews/ clean_fifteen_list.php>.

28. For much of my information on Ayurveda I am indebted to David Frawley's *Ayurvedic Healing: A Comprehensive Guide.* Delhi: Motilal Banarsidass Publishers, 2008 (1989). See p. 66.

29. Ibid., p. 79.

30. Ibid., pp. 100, 103.

31. Ibid., p. 55.

32. Carlos Castaneda. *The Teachings of Don Juan: A Yaqui Way of Knowledge*. Berkeley: University of California Press, (1968), p. 76.

33. CDC. "Obesity and Overweight" (data from 2011–2012) <http://www.cdc.gov/nchs/fastats/obesity-overweight.htm>.

34. ANAD. "Eating Disorder Statistics." <http://www.anad.org/get-information/about-eating-disorders/eating-disorders-statistics/>. Eating Disorder Coalition. "Facts About Eating Disorders: What the Research Shows." 2014 <http://www.eatingdisorderscoalition.org/documents/FactsAboutEatingDisorders2014.pdf>.

35. Laura Blue. "Being Overweight Is Linked to Lower Risk of Mortality," TIME.com, January 2, 2013 <http://healthland.time.com/2013/01/02/being-overweight-is-linked-to-lower-risk-of-mortality/>.

36. Thich Nhat Hanh. "Eating Together" <http://plumvillage.org/mindfulness-practice/eating-together/>.

37. Cesar Chavez. Quoted on the United States Farmworker Factsheet. Student Action with Farmworkers <https://saf-unite.org/content/united-states-farmworker-factsheet>.

38. For more information, see National Farm Worker Ministry, "Labor Laws" <http://nfwm.org/education-center/farm-worker-issues/labor-laws/>.

39. Southern Poverty Law Center. "Bandana Project to Spotlight Sexual Exploitation of Farmworker Women." 2009 <https://www.splcenter.org/news/2009/04/02/bandana-project-spotlight-sexual-exploitation-farmworker-women>.

40. See the National Farm Worker Ministry, "Union Label Shopping Guide." <http://nfwm.org/take-action/union-label-shopping-guide/>.

41. Human Rights Watch. "Blood, Sweat and Fear: Workers' Rights in U.S. Meat and Poultry Plants." January 24, 2005 <http://www.hrw.org/reports/2005/01/24/blood-sweat-and-fear>.

42. Ibid.

43. Ibid.

44. Jennifer Dillard. "A Slaughterhouse Nightmare: Psychological Harm Suffered by Slaughterhouse Employees and the Possibility of Redress through Legal Reform." *Georgetown Journal on Poverty Law & Policy* (2010) <http://papers.ssrn.com/sol3/papers.cfm?abstract_id=1016401>.

45. James McWilliams. "PTSD in the Slaughterhouse." *Texas Observer*, February 7, 2012 <http://www.texasobserver.org/ptsd-in-the-slaughterhouse/>.

46. World Cocoa Foundation. "Cocoa Market Update." March 2012 <http://worldcocoafoundation.org/wp-content/uploads/Cocoa-Market-Update-as-of-3.20.2012.pdf>.

47. David McKenzie and Brent Swails. "Child Slavery and Chocolate: All Too Easy to Find." CNN, January 19, 2012 <http://thecnnfreedomproject.blogs.cnn.com/2012/01/19/child-slavery-and-chocolate-all-too-easy-to-find/>.

48. Pratap Chatterjee. "Chocolate Slavery Case Against Nestlé Allowed to Proceed." *CorpWatch Blog*, December 24, 2013 <http://www.corpwatch.org/article.php?id=15915>.

49. Ibid.

50. International Labor Office of the International Programme on the Elimination of Child Labour (IPEC). "Combatting Child Labor in Cocoa Growing." 2005 <http://www.ilo.org/public//english/standards/ipec/themes/cocoa/download/2005_02_cl_cocoa.pdf>.

51. For example, see U.S. State Department. "Trafficking in Persons Report." June 12, 2007 <http://www.state.gov/documents/organization/82902.pdf>.

52. Food Empowerment Project. "Child Labor and Slavery in the Chocolate Industry." <http://www.foodispower.org/slavery-chocolate/>.

53. See <http://www.foodispower.org/chocolate-list/>.

54. Guy Lynn and Chris Rogers. "Civet Cat Coffee's Animal Cruelty Secrets." BBC News, September 13, 2013 <http://www.bbc.com/news/uk-england-london-24034029>.

55. National Resources Defense Council. "Coffee, Conservation, and Commerce in the Western Hemisphere: How Individuals and Institutions Can Promote Ecologically Sound Farming and Forest Management in Northern Latin America." <http://www.nrdc.org/health/farming/ccc/chap4.asp>.

56. Ibid.

57. Food Empowerment Project. "Bitter Brew: The Stirring Reality of Coffee." <http://www.foodispower.org/coffee/>.

58. World Health Organization. "Human Rights." <http://www.who.int/topics/human_rights/en/>.

59. Food Empowerment Project. "Food Deserts." <http://www.foodispower.org/food-deserts/>.

60. Bryan Walsh. "It's Not Just Genetics." *Time*, June 12, 2008.

61. Mari Gallagher. "Good Food: Examining the Impact of Food Deserts on Public Health in Chicago." Study commissioned by LaSalle Bank, 2006 <http://www.marigallagher. com/site_media/dynamic/project_files/1_ChicagoFoodDesertReport-Full.pdf>.

62. Miguel A. Altieri. "Modern Agriculture: Ecological Impacts and the Possibilities for Truly Sustainable Farming." Division of Insect Biology, University of California, Berkeley <http://nature.berkeley.edu/~miguel-alt/modern_agriculture.html> and Brenda Davis, R.D. and Vesanto Melina, M.S., R.D. *Becoming Vegan: The Complete Guide to Adopting a Healthy Plant-Based Diet*, Summertown, Tenn.: Book Publishing Co., 2000.

63. Roundtable on Sustainable Palm Oil. "Consumer Fact Sheet." <http://www.rspo.org/ consumers>.

64. Ibid.

65. Ibid.

66. Josephine Moulds and Emma Howard. "10 Things You Need to Know about Sustainable Palm Oil." *Guardian*, November 26, 2014 <http://www.theguardian.com/ sustainable-business/2014/nov/26/10-things-you-need-to-know-about-sustainable-palm-oil>.

Chapter 3: The Mind–Body Connection

1. Swami Satyananda Saraswati. *Asana Pranayama Mudra Bandha*. Bihar School of Yoga, India: Yoga Publications Trust, 2008 (1969), p. 12.

2. Ibid, p. 10.

3. Swami Satchidananda. "The Benefits of Hatha Yoga." <http://www.yogaville. org/2012/01/the-benefits-of-hatha-yoga>.

4. Swami Muktibodhananda. *Hatha Yoga Pradipika*. Bihar School of Yoga, India: Yoga Publications Trust, 2009 (1985), p. 186 (2:22).

Chapter 4: Cleansing the Soul

1. Martin Luther King Jr. *Strength to Love*. Minneapolis: Fortress Press, 2010, p. 47.

2. Blue Mountain Center of Meditation. "Passages for Meditation." <http://www. easwaran.org/the-dhammapada-twin-verses.html>.

3. See Swami Satchidananda, *Yoga Sutras*, p. 19 (1:13).

4. See Thich Nhat Hanh. *Old Path White Clouds: Walking in the Footsteps of the Buddha.* Berkeley: Parallax Press, 1991, pp. 483–484.

5. See Swami Satchidananda, *Yoga Sutras*, p. 82.

6. Quoted in *Divinity in Things: Religion without Myth* by Eric Ackroyd. Eastbourne, England: Sussex Academic Press, p. 60.

7. Translation by Sharon Gannon and David Life, cofounders of Jivamukti Yoga <http://jivamuktiyoga.com/teachings/focus-of-the-month/p/lokah-samastah-sukhino-bhavantu>.

8. Hanh, *Heart of the Buddha's Teaching*, pp. 156–157.

9. See Tsangnyon Heruka. *The Life of Milarepa.* New York: Penguin, 2010.

10. "Milarepa." Poet Seers <http://www.poetseers.org/spiritual-and-devotional-poets/buddhist/milarepa/>.

11. *maitri karuna mudita upekshanam sukha duhka punya apunya vishayanam bhavanatah chitta prasadanam).* Swami Satchidananda, *Yoga Sutras* (1:33).

12. Quoted by H. H. the Dalai Lama on the back cover of the tenth anniversary edition of *The Art of Happiness: A Handbook for Living.* New York: Riverhead Books, 1998.

13. Pema Chödrön. "Bodhichitta: The Excellence of Awakened Heart," Lion's Roar: Buddhist Wisdom for Our Time, September 1, 2001 <http://www.lionsroar.com/bodhichitta-the-excellence-of-awakened-heart/>.

14. Quoted in *The Harper Book of Quotations* (third edition) edited by Robert I. Fitzhenry. New York: HarperCollins, 1993, p. 356.

15. Hanh, *Heart of the Buddha's Teaching*, p. 9.

16. Swami Satchidananda. Quoted in "Daily Bread," Shanti Warrior Living Yoga, December 13, 2010 <http://www.shantiwarrior.com/dailybread.html/>.

17. This is a popular transliteration of a poem by Rumi. A more accurate translation is found in *Heart Yoga: The Sacred Marriage of Yoga and Mysticism* by Andrew Harvey and Karuna Erickson. Berkeley: North Atlantic Books, 2010, p. 66.

18. Quoted in Jamgön Kongtrül. *The Great Path of Awakening: The Classic Guide to Lojong, A Tibetan Buddhist Practice for Cultivating the Heart of Compassion.* Boston: Shambhala, 2005, p. 6.

19. See Harvey Alper. *Understanding Mantras.* New York: State University of New York, 1989, pp. 3–7.

20. Quoted in *Dhammapada* translated by Eknath Easwaran. Petaluma, Calif.: Nilgiri Press, 1985, p. 105.

21. Quoted in *Gandhi the Man: How One Man Changed Himself to Change the World* by Eknath Easwaran. Petaluma, Calif.: Nilgiri Press, p. 139.

22. *The Cloud of Unknowing* by James Walsh. Mahwah, N.J.: Paulist Press, p. 134.

23. Quoted in *Wisdom from World Religions: Pathways Toward Heaven on Earth* by John Marks Templeton. Radnor, Penn.: Templeton Foundation Press, p. 38.

24. Easwaran. *Bhagavad Gita*, p. 106 (3:19–32).

25. Hanh, *Heart of the Buddha's Teaching*, p. 140.

26. Easwaran, *Bhagavad Gita*, p. 177 (9:34).

27. Ibid., p. 62.

28. Leslie Goldman. "4 Amazing Health Benefits of Helping Others," *Huffington Post*, updated January 23, 2014 <http://www.huffingtonpost.com/2013/12/28/health-benefits-of-helping-others_n_4427697.html>.

29. Jeanie Lerche Davis. "The Science of Good Deeds" <http://www.webmd.com/balance/features/science-good-deeds>.

30. David McCleland and Carol Kirchnit. "The Effect of Motivational Arousal Through Films on Salivary Immunoglobulin A," *Psychology and Health* 2 (1988): 31–52.

31. Maria Pagano et al. "Helping Other Alcoholics in Alcoholics Anonymous and Drinking Outcomes: Findings from Project MATCH," *Journal of Studies on Alcohol* 65, no. 6 (2004): 766–773.

32. Stephen G. Post, Ph.D. "It's Good to Be Good: Science Says It's So," *Health Progress*, July–August 2009 <http://www.stonybrook.edu/bioethics/goodtobegood.pdf>.

33. Ibid.

34. Allan Luks. "Helper's High: Volunteering Makes People Feel Good, Physically and Emotionally," *Psychology Today* 22, no. 10 (October 1988): 34–42.

35. Dacher Keltner. "The Compassionate Instinct," Greater Good: The Science of a Meaningful Life, University of California, Berkeley, March 1, 2004 <http://greatergood.berkeley.edu/article/item/the_compassionate_instinct>.

36. Thich Nhat Hanh. Quoted in the transcript for "On Being with Krista Tippett," January 22, 2015 <http://www.onbeing.org/program/thich-nhat-hanh-mindfulness-suffering-and-engaged-buddhism/transcript/7234>.

37. Stephen G. Post, "It's Good to Be Good."

38. Ibid.

39. Easwaran, *Bhagavad Gita*, p. 108 (3:35).

Chapter 5: A Practical Manual for Living One Step at a Time

1. Swami Satchidananda, *Yoga Sutras*, p. 146 (2:42).

2. See Thich Nhat Hanh, *Understanding Our Mind: 50 Verses on Buddhist Psychology*. Berkeley: Parallax Press, 2006, pp. 150–153.

3. Edward O. Wilson: *Biophilia: The Human Bond with Other Species*. Harvard: Harvard University Press, 2003 (1984).

4. Erich Fromm. *The Heart of Man*. New York: American Mental Health Foundation, 2010 (1964), p. 9.

5. National Institutes of Health, NIH in the News. "The Power of Love Hugs and Cuddles Have Long-Term Effects." February 2007 <http://newsinhealth.nih.gov/2007/February/docs/01features_01.htm>.

6. Blue Mountain Center of Meditation. "You Are That." <http://www.easwaran.org/the-chandogya-upanishad-you-are-that.html>.

7. See WWF <http://www.worldwildlife.org/threats/deforestation>.

8. U.S. Fish & Wildlife Service. *2011 National Survey of Fishing, Hunting, and Wildlife-Associated Recreation*, p. 4. <https://www.census.gov/prod/2012pubs/fhw11-nat.pdf>.

9. U.S. Department of Agriculture. "Organic Production." <http://www.ers.usda.gov/data-products/organic-production/documentation.aspx>.

10. Matthew Scully. *Dominion: The Power of Man, the Suffering of Animals, and the Call to Mercy*. New York: St. Martin's, 2002.

11. David Frawley, *Ayurvedic Healing*.

12. Harvard Health Letter. "Spending Time Outdoors Is Good for You." July 2010 <http://www.health.harvard.edu/press_releases/spending-time-outdoors-is-good-for-you>.

13. Jean-Jacques Rousseau, *The Basic Political Writings*. Translated by Donald Cress. Indianapolis: Hackett Publishing Company, 1987, p. 19.

14. Swami Satchidananda, *Yoga Sutras*, p. 84 (2:3).

15. Ibid., p. 86 (2:5).

16. Hanh, *Heart of the Buddha's Teaching*, p. 24.

17. A version of this story is told in *Being Peace* by Thich Nhat Hanh and Jack Kornfield. Berkeley: Parallax Press, p. 68.

18. Pema Chödrön's version is in *Start Where You Are: A Guide to Compassionate Living*. Boston: Shambhala, 1994, pp. 48–49.

19. Swami Satchidananda, *Yoga Sutras*, p. 127 (2:33).

20. Blue Mountain Center of Meditation. "Passages for Meditation." <http://www. easwaran.org/the-dhammapada-twin-verses.html>.

21. MyPlate is available at the USDA's website <http://www.choosemyplate.gov/>.

Conclusion

1. Quoted in Hanh, *Heart of the Buddha's Teaching*, p. 15. ❁

ॐ
Acknowledgments

I believe there is a deep reverence, wisdom, and love within the heart of all beings, but we don't discover that on our own. And we can't cultivate that enlightened heart without nurturing and support from the world in which we live. I am eternally and infinitely grateful to all of my kind, wise, loving teachers, friends, and family (human and non-human) who have helped me to see the interconnection of all life, to discover my own love for all beings, and to live a life that manifests that understanding and love as best as I know how at the moment. I can't possibly name all those to whom I'm indebted because every being we ever encounter has some effect on us in some way: for example, my friend Ernesto in middle school, whose last name I can't even remember now. He told me one day while we were riding the bus home from school that I was the kindest person in school. When he said it, my heart sank because I knew that, in truth, I was not nearly as kind as he thought. I had recently picked on one of our classmates, and I absolutely tormented my poor parents throughout my adolescence. I didn't deserve Ernesto's high praise, but he saw something good in me and that recognition motivated me to be better. We all influence each other. A butterfly flaps her wings in Peru, and the weather in Antarctica is affected.

I'm thankful for the conditions and circumstances that I was born into that have allowed me the health and freedom to wander onto this path, to speak my mind, to live from my heart. This book wouldn't have come into existence if not for all the brave, smart, kind, patient, and non-judgmental animal rights heroes I've met along the way who have mentored me, educated me, and inspired me, whether they knew

227

it or not. There are too many to name, but I at least need to mention those who initially introduced me to the truth and who are responsible for my own awakening: Mindy Kursban, Dawn Moncrief, Alex Hershaft, Erica Meier, Paul Shapiro, Terry Cummings, Dave Hoerauf, Jon Camp, Lynda Cozart, Tracy Silverman, all the volunteers at Poplar Spring—including Deb Durant and Ryan MacMichael—all the wonderful people who've worked at Compassion Over Killing, and the many other inspiring volunteers, like my friend Simone Guarani-Kaiowa de Lima.

All these activists and many others who dedicate their lives to helping alleviate the suffering of our non-human kin were the first bodhisattvas I ever met, and I continue to feed on and be inspired by the selflessness and compassion I see in my activist friends today. These include all the ARC group and beyond (Anjie, Jeff, Veronica, Roy, Joanie, John, Linda, Debbie, Susan, Lella, Tymber, Jarrod, Chelsey, Ryan, Baby Lucy, Kim and Kim, Karen, Ali, Heather, Steven, MaryAnn, Roz, Mark, Thomas, and Yuri), and all my other compassionate friends around the globe who inspire me constantly, all of them the truest karma yogis, most of who don't even know that's what they are.

I offer deep bows to all the spiritual teachers who helped me find the tools to ground my activism in Gandhian principles of non-violence; to stay connected to my own compassion; and to learn how not to give in to the forces of anger or depression that are such a natural response to a world filled with so much injustice and suffering. I extend my deepest gratitude to the teachers who live the radical compassion taught by the Buddha: Thank you, Ven. Thich Nhat Hanh, Dr. Will Tuttle, Ven Tashi Nyima, Brother Stream, Sister Pine, Sister Boi Ngiem, and all the other monastics at Magnolia Grove and Plum Village. When I traveled to India in 2010, I had no idea how much my life would change. I didn't quite know what I was doing or what I was looking for, but I trusted that I would get what I needed, and I couldn't have been more fortunate than I was to find my teachers there: Sri Man, Sanjay Naithany, Roshan, and a very special dog named Shanti. Thank you to all of the teachers and community at Yogaville who so embody the teachings of Sri Swami Satchidananda, including Bhagavan Metro, Prakasha Capen, Katherine Lakshmi Sendall, Stacy

Kamala Waltman, and the rest of the community of teachers and students from whom I've learned so much about living yoga.

To everyone who helped me directly with this book, whose insights and ideas are inextricably interwoven throughout—especially, my first editors Katherine Lakshmi Sendall and Sylvia Glover (a.k.a. Mom) for the invaluable help and better judgment than my own, in addition to your loving support and belief in me. Thank you, Kara Davis, for such a broad vision and intelligence and the opportunity to expand and improve on the first draft of this book that came across your desk. And to Martin Rowe, for offering a forum where books like this one—books that aim to improve the world at least a little—are given a chance; for pulling this book together into a much more cohesive and readable whole; and for believing in the message of the book.

I thank all the brave, compassionate activists in the world collecting and disseminating information so that we all can see the truth and make choices that help alleviate suffering. Without the activists who put together the early PETA undercover videos I may never have opened my eyes. Without the brave activists who filmed the Chinese fur-farming videos, as well as my dog Penelope, I may never have found the motivation I needed to go vegan.

To Scott, for helping me find the path, and surrender to it, as well as teaching me how to love another human unconditionally.

Many thanks to Ginger Graf Dunaway for giving me the opportunity to teach yoga in the way that is most authentic for me and for creating such a beautiful sanctuary to do it in. Thank you to John Gulas for creating a kirtan community in Mobile, Alabama, that feeds all of us in so many ways and to all the yogis and musicians who come through town sharing the teachings and practice of bhakti yoga, the yoga of love—especially the friends who keep coming back and whose lives are such a beautiful manifestation of the teachings—like Rahaysa and Prema Hara.

Thanks to Valerie Mitchell for endless patience and making it fun to take pictures, and to Renee Hoadley and Jordan Laughlin for being such beautiful human beings in addition to such beautiful yoga models.

Special thanks to Surf Dog, Bubby, and Tippy—my non-human family—who remind me daily how deserving all non-humans are of love and respect, how unique each individual is, and for helping me connect with my own highest Self, which is love and compassion, joy and selflessness.

Nothing good I've ever done would have been possible without my open-minded, tenderhearted, ever-supportive parents, who both defied the odds and went vegan over the age of sixty. My crazy dad Joe, who himself learned love from non-humans, who raised me to see all that creeps and crawls and slithers and swims and walks on four legs with the eyes of mercy and compassion, from whom I inherited a heart that feels the pain of all creatures. And my mom, Sylvia—gentle, joyful, silly, brave, and effortlessly kind to all beings—who is the constant voice in my ear telling me I am loved. ❀

ॐ
Glossary of Terms

ahimsa, non-harm, non-violence

ajna, the sixth, or third-eye *chakra*

aparigraha, non-greed

asana, physical posture

asmita, over-identification with the ego

Ashtanga, a vigorous system of yoga developed by Sri K. Pattabhi Jois

asteya, non-stealing

atha, now

Atman, Divine Self

avatar, incarnation

avidya, ignorance

Ayurveda, the ancient Hindu system of healing

baba, term of affection used for holy man or saint

Basti, washing and toning the large intestine

Bhakti, devotion

bodhicitta, awakened heart and mind

bodhisattva, enlightened beings who help release others from misery

brahmacharya, celibacy

brahmin, priest

chakra, a wheel, an energy vortex in the body

dharana, one-pointed concentration

Dharma, the core of the Buddha's teachings

dhauti, internal cleaning

doshas, forces

dhyana, meditation

duhkha, pain

gunas, qualities in *Ayurveda*

hatha, union of life force with mental energy

ida nadi, negative flow of energy in the body

ishvara pranidhana, total surrender to the Divine

jnana, wisdom

kapalbhathi, breathing technique to purify the frontal region of the brain

Kapha, one of the three basic *doshas* in *Ayurveda*

karma, action

karuna, compassion

kirtan, call-and-response style of singing used in yoga

klesha, mental obstacle

kriyas, cleansing practices

magga, the path to the cessation of suffering

maha, great

maitri, loving kindness

manas, mental

mantra, a chant or saying used in meditation

maya, veil of ignorance and illusion

mudita, joy

mudra, symbolic hand gesture

muladhara, the first, or root, *chakra*

nadis, energy channels in the body

nadi shodhan, alternate-nostril breathing

nauli, massaging and strengthening the abdominal organs

neti, purifying the nasal passages

nirodha, cessation

nirvana, enlightenment

niyamas, ethical prescriptions

om, the originating sound of the universe

pingala nadi, positive flow of energy in the body

Pitta, one of the three basic *doshas* in *Ayurveda*

prana, universal energy, breath

pranayama, breath control

pratipaksha bhavana, replacing the disturbing force with a positive one

pratyahara, sense withdrawal

raga, pleasure

raja, royal

rajasic, a quality of mind in *Ayurveda*

rishi, sage

sadhana, range of spiritual practices, including meditation and scriptural study

sahasrara, the seventh, or crown *chakra*

samadhi, spiritual absorption, or union with the Divine

Samkhya, one of six orthodox schools of Indian philosophy related to yoga and *Ayurveda*

samskaras, deep unconscious mental impressions that create habits

samudāya, the origin of suffering

sankalpa, intention, resolution

santosha, contentment

sattvic, a quality of mind in *Ayurveda*

satya, honesty, truth

saucha, purity in mind, speech, and body

shakti, energy

shanti, peace

shashankasana, the rabbit pose in yoga

shatkarma, six cleansing practices

sushumna nadi, main energy channel of body

svadhyaya, study of the Divine Self

tamasic, a quality of mind in *Ayurveda*

tapas, heat

Tonglen, a Buddhist meditation practice

trataka, intense gazing at an object

ujjayi, a breathing technique

upeksha, equanimity

vanara, monkey-like person

Vajrayana, a school of Buddhism

Vata, one of the three basic *doshas* in *Ayurveda*

Vedas, the seminal Indian spiritual texts

vinyasa, a style of yoga in which movement is coordinated with the breath.

yamas, ethical proscriptions

yoga, union; or a spiritual, mental, and physical discipline

yoga nidra, form of deep, guided meditation

yogasana, the posture suited to meditation

Yuga, an Age of time ✸

About the Author

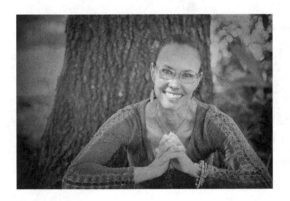

Tracey Winter Glover, J.D., graduated phi beta kappa from the University of Michigan and holds a law degree from the University of Michigan's law school. She practiced law in Washington D.C. for eight years before heading to Rishikesh, India to study yoga and meditation. Since returning from India, she has been running a vegan meal delivery business in Mobile, Alabama, as well as teaching yoga and training yoga teachers through her yoga school Shanti Warrior Living Yoga. In 2014, she cofounded Awakening Respect and Compassion for All Sentient Beings (ARC), a nonprofit dedicated to raising awareness about the impact of our daily choices on other species and the environment and creating a more sustainable and compassionate world for all sentient beings. ❀

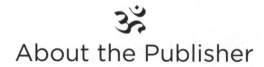

About the Publisher

LANTERN BOOKS was founded in 1999 on the principle of living with a greater depth and commitment to the preservation of the natural world. In addition to publishing books on animal advocacy, vegetarianism, religion, and environmentalism, Lantern is dedicated to printing books in the U.S. on recycled paper and saving resources in day-to-day operations. Lantern is honored to be a recipient of the highest standard in environmentally responsible publishing from the Green Press Initiative. ❈

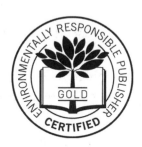

lanternbooks.com